JASON VALE'S

Super Juice Me!

28-DAY JUICE PLAN

While the author of this book has made every effort to ensure that the information contained in this book is as accurate and up-to-date as possible at the time of publication, medical and pharmaceutical knowledge is constantly changing and the application of it to particular circumstances depends on many factors. This book should not be used as an alternative to specialist medical advice and it is recommended that readers always consult a qualified medical profession for individual advice before following any new diet or health programme. The author and the publishers cannot be held responsible for any errors and omissions that can be found in the text, or any actions that may be taken by a reader, as a result of any reliance on the information contained in the text, which are taken entirely at the reader's own risk.

First published in 2015 by Juice Master Publications.

ISBN 978-0-95-476645-0

Copyright © Jason Vale & Juice Master Publications 2015

Written by Jason Vale with acknowledged contributions.

Design & layout by Light Mill Media LLP

CONTENTS

THANK YOU

I would like to thank the people who helped to make this book possible. This doesn't simply include those who have helped with the layout, proof-reading and so on, but those at Juicy HQ who help to make a difference to so many every day. These include: John Pickering, Andrea Wells, Kirsty Heber-Smitg, Nina Chauhan, Daniel and Sarah Gresly, Joanna Comber, Oliver Saunders, Tom Nicholson and Skye Lyselle. I would like to say a special thank you to Alex and Charlie Leith, two people who I have had the great fortune of working with for over a decade and the people who made *Super Juice Me!* The Movie possible. Without the film and the huge impact it has had around the world, this book wouldn't be here, so THANK YOU Alex and Charlie for helping to spread the word in so many ways and for being the incredibly special people you are.

...and lastly, but most importantly, I'd like to thank my rock Katie. They say that behind every good man is a great great woman and that statement couldn't be truer than here. Katie you are my world and I cannot thank you enough for all you do. You are a truly amazing woman and I am blessed to have you share your life with little ole me, I LOVE YOU! x

This book is dedicated to my beautiful mother

NINA BARBARA VALE

I cannot believe that the one person in the world I want to read this book, never actually will. My mother was my everything. Words simply cannot and will not ever do justice to what this amazing, kind, beautiful, generous, loving, caring and all-round top woman meant to me and the people around her. Words also cannot and will not ever truly explain the gaping hole in my world now she's gone. It has been four years, to the day as I write this very page, since she left, and it feels like yesterday.

Everyone says their mother is special, but if you'd ever had the good fortune of knowing Nina you would know that every now and then the world produces a very, very special kind of person. I had the remarkably good fortune of having her as my mother, father, best friend, brother and sister for 41 years of my life. We were inseparable and would speak on the phone for at least an hour a day. I still cannot bring myself to delete her numbers from my mobile phone and can barely, even today, look at a picture of her. I watched a film the other day in which someone, when explaining why they didn't talk about the passing of a certain relative, said, 'I guess some things are just too big to talk about'. What I am writing now is perhaps the most I have ever really talked about my mother's passing. It's also the hardest page to write in the whole book.

One day I will write a full report of what happened to my

mother. I will explain how she was misdiagnosed for four years and why I believe my mother would be alive today, if that misdiagnosis hadn't happened. But now is not the time.

I write this dedication for two reasons. One is to let everyone reading this book know that I would have achieved nothing without my mother. If any of my previous books has helped you in any way, it's down ultimately to this extraordinary woman. The other is because of what happened to her. The aim of this book is to inspire you to do something about your health before it's too late. We all think we are invincible until the unthinkable happens, and by then it may even be too late.

My mother told me in late January 2010 that she had stage 4 lung cancer and had been given six months to live. Not all cancers are the same and stage 1 breast cancer is not, in real terms, the same disease as stage 4 lung cancer. Her cancer was very aggressive and she passed just eight months after her diagnosis. The biggest tragedy is that she had gone to her doctor *four years* prior to being diagnosed with stage 4 lung cancer, only to be to told she had chronic obstructive pulmonary disease (COPD) and was given an asthma pump. As it turns out, although asthma pumps are great for treating the symptoms of asthma, they do nothing for lung cancer! I honestly believe that if my mother had been properly diagnosed she would still be here today.

I am not suggesting for one second that any of the information in this book is a 'cure' for any cancer, so please never misread or misquote what I am saying. What I strongly believe, though, is that if my mother had been correctly diagnosed she, with the help of nature's finest nutritional 'medicine', would have at least had a fighting chance. The earlier you detect any disease the more chance you have of treating it successfully. Four years of constant misdiagnoses meant the cancer was free to spread and it was just too late.

This book is designed to help people take control of their health *before* anything truly horrific happens, in other words *before* it's too late. This book/plan is designed with *common lifestyle diseases* in mind and, as I will explain in depth in the book, it's not a 'cure' for anything. Having said that, many people who have experienced the *Super Juice Me!* programme have seen truly extraordinary results and often use the word 'cure' (feel free to flick to the centre colour pages to get a quick glimpse of what just 28 days of good nutrition can do for many different illnesses).

If I could turn the clock back I would. I think of almost nothing else some days. I think about how this programme, if it had been implemented at the right time, would have, in my opinion, made a fundamental difference to my mother's outcome. I wish every day that I'd taken more control of her health way before she was even diagnosed. The warning signals were there, even though the doctors missed them time and time again. My mother would have felt them, but ignored them or dismissed them as *'nothing to overly worry about because the doctor said so'*. I feel we can often sense when something isn't quite right.

If you are not *'feeling quite right'* or you are suffering from a lifestyle disease and medical drugs just aren't working, then I am pleased you have picked up this book. Now you have it in your hands, I sincerely hope you read it and do the full *28-Day Juice Plan*. Even if you don't feel any different at the end, it's only fruit and vegetables and you won't have done any further harm. At least you have to give yourself a fighting chance by trying it.

As mentioned, I will document my mother's full story one day, but this isn't the time. My beautiful mother only ever wanted to try and help people. That was her default, and she would go without to make sure another person was taken care of. To say she was unique is to do her a disservice. She was the most loving, giving, caring, incredible woman I have ever had the good fortune of knowing. I hope her caring comes through in this book via me. It's a cliché to say *'If this book helps just one person then it would have been worth it'*, but that is how I genuinely feel and I sincerely hope you are that one person.

Nina Barbara Vale, my life changed the second you left and will never be the same again – see you on the other side kid…

BEFORE WE BEGIN...

READ THIS BIT...

Let me introduce myself...

My name is Jason Vale and I'm often otherwise known as, 'The Juice Master'. I am the first to acknowledge it's a ridiculous 'aka', but it wasn't of my doing and came about years ago as a result of the film *Pulp Fiction*. It's a long story and I won't bore you with it here, but I felt the need for you to know that I am not a self-proclaimed 'Juice Master'!

I have been teaching and writing about juicing for rapid healthy weight loss and optimum health for well over a decade. During this time I have had the privilege of seeing tens of thousands of people from all walks of life all over the world improve their health and well-being with the help of freshly extracted juice.

By simply using the freshly extracted organic liquid fuel contained within nature's finest fruits and vegetables and removing the rubbish coming into the body, I have seen almost every common ailment either improve dramatically or be cured altogether. I cannot possibly understate the healing effect freshly extracted juice can have on both the body and mind, when done in the correct way.

If you have *almost any common ailment or lifestyle disease* and follow this **28-Day Super Juice Me! Juice Plan** to the letter, the chances are you will see quite extraordinary results.

However, before we begin, I wish to make my qualifications clear:

I AM NOT A DOCTOR

I am, however, someone who has studied *juice therapy* for

over twelve years and I have witnessed first hand the positive health benefits it has had, not only in my own life, but also in the lives of the tens of thousands of people I hear from every year. I have read thousands of books on the subject of juicing, nutrition and addiction, and I have now written eleven books in the area of addiction, juicing and health myself. I have also attended well over a thousand lectures on the subject.

On a personal health level, I spent many years living with psoriasis, a chronic skin condition. I was covered from head to toe in the disease and, for most of the winter months, couldn't wear jeans without my skin cracking. It covered nearly every inch of my body, including my face. I also suffered from asthma. This condition was so bad I would need to take the blue inhaler up to 14 times a day and the brown inhaler (the steroid based one) once a day. I also had extremely bad eczema covering the backs of my knees, which would crack, bleed and ooze pus.

On top of these conditions, hay fever also affected my life. Like many diseases, there is a spectrum of symptom severity – which I will cover later – and hay fever is one in which this spectrum is extremely wide. There are some who get slightly itchy eyes and mild sinus problems. Others have hay fever so badly that they can barely breathe and cannot move or work. That was me. It is a shame they still call this condition 'hay fever', as severe hay fever is rarely, if ever, taken seriously. Yet the sufferer can be confined to their home or have to spend time in air-conditioned buildings for days to receive any kind of respite.

I was also overweight and had my fair share of problems with food, alcohol, nicotine and marijuana addiction.

I spent many, many years researching my own conditions in order to find natural treatments as conventional medicine had completely failed me. I studied addiction intensely and once I had conquered my own, I ran an addiction clinic for years helping others. So, although I am not a doctor, I have well over a decade's worth of experience in the field of nutrition and the natural *'alternative'* treatments for disease.

It may be worth pointing out very early in this book, in case you feel a doctor would be much more qualified to advise you in this area than I am, that the average doctor in the UK will spend just three to six hours studying nutrition in the entire *six years* of their medical training. That's just three to six hours, yes *hours*.

This I still find hard to believe, but it is perfectly true. It becomes even harder to believe when you think that, according to the World Health Organization, eighty-five per cent of all disease in western society is as a direct result of what we put into our mouths. Yet our medical profession will spend only around three hours studying the very things which are known to cause the vast *majority* of *lifestyle* diseases. Diseases they are treating every single day of their professional lives.

I AM NOT ANTI DOCTOR OR ANTI PHARMA

I also wish to make something else clear. Although I teach natural juice therapy, and therefore am often put into the 'alternative' or 'complementary' medicine camp, I am not against the medical profession. Far from it in fact.

You will read later that, at times, for many diseases *short-term* medical intervention and, *at times*, long-term medical intervention are vital. It can be dangerous to dismiss all conventional medicine, as some people do. For now though, I need you to know I am not a doctor in any sense of the word. It appears these days you can simply hop on a plane to the USA, do a very short course in almost anything and, bingo, you're a 'doctor'. As far as I am concerned, the only people I feel who should be able to use the term doctor, are *medically trained* doctors. We then should have different prefixes and terms for those who have studied incredibly hard in other areas to earn their particular 'doctorate'. There is a funny scene in the US hit sitcom *Friends*, where the character Ross walks into a hospital and says to a nurse who asks his name, 'I'm Dr Ross Geller.' To which his friend Rachael replies, 'Shuuush, Ross, that actually means something in here.' Ross had his doctorate in palaeontology, and knowledge of dinosaurs isn't particularly useful when someone is having a heart attack! We are in a world where I could, if I wanted to, call myself 'The Juice Doctor'. But that would be somewhat misleading.

Because I am not a doctor and because the pure, organic, nutrient-rich liquid fuel found in all plant foods is not recognized as medicine in any way shape or form, (because the world is run by Big Business and Big Pharma and not by natural common sense) I need to make the following statement:

PLEASE CONSULT YOUR DOCTOR BEFORE YOU EMBARK ON THIS 28-DAY 'SUPER JUICE ME!' JUICE PLAN

...and please can I add...

PLEASE <u>DO NOT</u> COME OFF ANY MEDICATION WITHOUT CONSULTING YOUR DOCTOR FIRST

There – covered!

This doesn't mean I don't believe that many doctors aren't qualified to help in the area of nutrition either. Without doubt, many are. I just wanted to point out what many don't know: the *average* doctor spends just three to six hours of their six years of medical training on nutrition. Some go on to study this area after they have qualified, but many do not, and many, if they have studied it at all, will be teaching out-of-date theories in this area. I will repeat this point over and over again: I am *not* anti-doctor or against *all* pharmaceuticals. I believe I would have been dead I without my asthma pump. What I am against is the pill-popping frenzy which is taking place for many, many conditions that could easily be treated by natural means.

I would also like to point out two other things before we start our juicing journey to optimum health together.

I AM NOT A SCIENTIST

I do not purport to be a scientist or to have any scientific background. This doesn't mean that this juice plan isn't based on a degree of science, because it is. However, I simply want to be 100 per cent transparent and say that although I see the need for some science, science is not all it's cracked up to be. Often what is deemed to be 'scientific fact' is in reality nothing more than 'scientific hypothesis'.

Let us not forget that according to the 'best scientific minds' in the world global disaster was going to prevail immediately the clocks struck midnight at the beginning of the year 2000. If you recall, we had a constant diet of scary news reports telling us that planes would fall out of the sky, that economic meltdown was on the horizon because banks' computers wouldn't recognize the year 2000 and so on. There was even a BUG WATCH on UK TV, running an entire live update on the disaster as it unfolded, very similar to election night on TV.

And what actually happened in the end? Nothing! Scientific evidence 'proved' that unless action was taken (at the cost of $300 billion, it's worth adding – that's THREE HUNDRED BILLION DOLLARS!) disaster would happen. Governments believed their scientists to such an extent that they spent millions of pounds of *our* tax money trying to prevent the disaster. And in case you feel *'it's better to be safe than sorry'* (which is usually the excuse we hear for the often outrageous misuse of public money), countries which spent no money at all trying to prevent the 'millennium bug' received the same fate as us – nothing! As you can imagine it made for a riveting all-night live TV show as the non-news came rolling in.

Fear can be used to justify almost anything, no matter how ridiculous, including the massive over-use and catastrophic misuse of medical drugs. You can after all justify the spending of almost any amount of money on the 'war on disease'.

In the film *Super Juice Me!* many people, including myself, challenge some of the 'science' to do with conventional medicine. I point out how easy it is to 'prove' or make a very good case for your hypothesis – especially if you just happen to be a drug company with billions of dollars to throw at finding a positive result.

The swine flu debacle that occurred in 2009 was another classic example of 'science fact' becoming 'science fiction'. The British government spent over £1 BILLION stockpiling anti-viral drugs such as Tamiflu and ordered enough vaccines to give two doses to every man, woman and child.

The Chief Medical Officer, no less, predicted 65,000 people could die of the virus, putting the very fabric of society at risk. In the end just over 400 people died in the UK as a result of swine flu. More than 80 per cent of them already had underlying health issues. That means fewer than 100 people were killed by swine flu alone, not 65,000 as predicted!

I think the worst part of this particular health debacle was how the government put unqualified people in call centres to diagnose and dispense medication. If I diagnosed one person and prescribed them a medical drug I would find myself in prison! However, when the government does it, it appears to be 'for the greater good'.

In the end it came out that some people who were directly responsible for advising the mass use of certain anti-viral drugs had financial links to the drug companies supplying them. It is also worth pointing out that in Poland the government refused to be frightened into taking such drastic action, and just 150 people died because of swine flu in a country with a population of over 40 million. It is also worth pointing out that this number is roughly the same as the number of those who would have died of 'normal' flu.

The difference between Poland and the UK was nothing...

other than that the UK government spent £1 billion and the Polish government didn't!

The final point I wish to make before you dive into what I hope will prove to be an incredibly life-changing experience for you is that...

I AM NOT A NUTRITIONIST
AND
I AM NOT A DIETICIAN

You may not know this, but anyone, and I do mean *anyone*, can at the time of writing this book legally call themselves a nutritionist. Many 'nutritionists' give the whole industry an incredibly bad name and it gives ammunition to people like Ben Goldacre, author of the genuinely very good books *Bad Science* and *Bad Pharma*, to hammer the entire industry. Other people may have called me a nutritionist, but I have never actually called myself one (well not knowingly anyway). If anything I am a natural juice therapist and a health adviser or health and addictions coach, although I don't like any of those terms either. What I am definitely not is a 'dietician'.

Unlike the title 'nutritionist', only a qualified person can call him or herself a dietician. It takes around six years of intensive study to become one of those. Most dieticians have excellent knowledge of how the human body works, what you should eat and drink for optimum health, what the difference between 'healthy weight', 'overweight' and 'obese' is, and what the right level of exercise is for you...*according to what they've been taught that is.*

And therein lies the problem. If what they are being taught is simply not true or is based on out-of-date thinking they may not always be the best people to learn from. For example, take the BMI (Body Mass Index) as an example. This is a *'scientific'* index that is used as standard practice by the medical profession to see if someone is in the healthy weight range, overweight range or obese range. According to this 'scientific' scale Brad Pitt is overweight and Johnny Wilkinson (the very lean rugby player) is *'obese!'* This is because this antiquated system doesn't take muscle mass into the equation.

Just because it is science and is being taught by someone who has government-recognized qualifications, this doesn't make it right. There have been thousands of cases of dieticians and doctors teaching things in the area of health that have later proved to be completely wrong, yet at the time these claims were made with utter certainty. One classic example is that of doctors advertising cigarettes on television and encouraging patients to smoke to *'calm them down'*. Yes, doctors once suggested that a known stimulant was a way to calm people down. This seems outrageous now, especially the advertising of cigarettes on TV, but it was deemed good medical advice in some circumstances at the time.

At the present time, doctors prescribe antibiotics left right and centre to treat colds and flu, even though it is now known that antibiotics do nothing to kill a virus, they only work on bacteria.

What I describe today as 'The Great Cholesterol Mistake' will be tomorrow's 'what we have learnt now is...' moment.

Just the word *cholesterol* is enough to send a shiver down the average spine. Yet despite what you may think, the 'high cholesterol equals heart disease' mantra is not a fact, it's a hypothesis. The fact that there is usually more cholesterol present in someone with heart disease doesn't mean that the high cholesterol is the cause of the heart disease.

One of the fundamental rules of science is this: *association does not automatically equate to causation.* This means that just because a certain factor, such as high cholesterol, is frequently observed in heart disease patients, this doesn't mean it actually causes the disease. In 1957 John Yudkin published a study showing that TV and radio ownership were far more closely associated with coronary mortality in England than any dietary factor. Despite the strength of Yudkin's correlation, we know that televisions and radios do not cause heart disease. No one seriously believes that if we were to ditch our radios and TVs it would grant us instant immunity from heart disease! It's the same with high cholesterol and heart disease: the high cholesterol could be *secondary*. I am not saying that it is secondary. I am just saying that this subject needs to be studied a lot more before we start handing out cholesterol-lowering drugs to all and sundry. Timothy Noakes, Professor of Exercise and Sports Science at the University of Cape Town, South Africa, says, 'Focusing on an elevated blood cholesterol concentration as the exclusive cause of coronary heart disease is unquestionably the worst medical error of our time. After reviewing all the scientific evidence, I draw just one conclusion: never prescribe a statin drug for a loved one'.

Cholesterol lowering drugs have now become one of the pharmaceutical industry's biggest earners, bringing *billions* (not millions) into their coffers each year, usually at the taxpayer's expense here in the UK. At the time of writing this book, statins are being recommended for *healthy* patients when their risk of heart disease is greater than 20 per cent over 10 years. The proposal is to drop that to ten per cent. According to the doctors' magazine *Pulse* this could increase the number of healthy Britons on statins to 12 million. That's 12 million perfectly healthy people who have just a 10 per cent chance of heart disease being given liver-toxic drugs *for life*. The medical profession and science have been wrong in the past and I believe they are very wrong about statins. Time will tell, but watch this space. 'The Great Cholesterol Mistake' will be making headlines one day for sure.

THE BIG FAT MISTAKE

In terms of diet though, I feel there has been no bigger mistake made by qualified, state-registered, government-backed dieticians and doctors than the 'anti-fat' debacle. This went on for years and, sadly, the 'Fat makes you fat and is the root of all evil' mantra is still believed by the vast majority of people even today. Fat, it turns out, is not the evil substance that makes you fat and causes heart disease after all. No, it's white refined sugar and its derivatives that are unquestionably the culprits, not the big F. I wrote about this in my very first book, *Slim For Life... Freedom From The Food Trap* and was hammered for making such an outrageous statement.

There are far, far too many examples of how scientific 'facts' are no more than hypotheses or are even completely wrong. Alone they could fill the entire book, which clearly we don't have room for. I have added these few examples in order to start the book with an open and free mind, free and open to a new way of looking at how many lifestyle diseases can and should, be treated. You have, I am guessing, picked up this book with one purpose in mind: to do something once and for all about your weight and state of health. There will of course be some of those reading this now who have picked it up merely to pick holes, but the majority of you need help with your health, and you are the ones I am interested in. For this book to have the effect you desire, there are three starting instructions you must adhere to:

1. READ THE BOOK
2. READ THE BOOK
3. READ THE BOOK

This is an instruction I have in all of my books and it's probably more important in this one than in any of the others. This is a full 28-Day 'juice only' plan and you cannot underestimate the importance of being fully prepared *before* you start. Getting the right juicer and so on is one part of it, but it's far from being the most important part. I would say, after 15 years' experience in this field, that getting fully mentally prepared is the single most important factor. It can easily be the difference between success and failure. Everything you need to know to successfully complete the programme is in the book; so please:

DO NOT START UNTIL YOU HAVE READ
THIS BABY FROM COVER TO COVER

Right, now the introduction and all the disclaimers are out of the way, let's crack on...

No wait ...

HOLD THE FIRST PAGE...
NEWS JUST IN!

This morning, and half-way through writing this book, I received an email about someone who has just competed the *Super Juice Me! 28-Day Juice Plan*. It's the sort of email that stops you in your tracks and reminds you of why you are doing what you're doing. It's the type of email which enables you to rise above the sceptics and solidify your confidence in the message you are spreading. I have included it now at the very start, in order to illustrate just how big an effect this programme can have on someone's life on every level. I am hoping it will inspire you to read the rest of the book and change your life by getting 'Super Juiced' yourself. This is the email which was forwarded onto me by the lovely Nina in the office just now:

I hope you don't mind me messaging you but I wanted to let you know about a friend of mine who has just completed the *28-Day juice plan*. See over years of encouraging people to juice, lots have taken to it and been inspired to keep going with it. So yes it's a big deal but maybe not that much of a big deal compared to my friend Lee. You see Lee lost his brother at the age of 14; he is 31 now and lives with his parents. He turned to alcohol and cocaine and spent up to £1000 a week on this habit. A complete downward spiral. No one thought Lee would get off it unless he went to rehab or some drastic action. But after years' worth of patience and talking with him, he messaged me one day and said I need to buy a juicer what one shall I get. So I advised him, then a couple of days later, he messages me and says ok I've started, so far I have squirted lime in my eye and nearly cut my finger! I was so proud of him that he took that action. Then when he told me he was doing the 28-Day one, well I nearly fainted!

He completed it yesterday and lost 2 stone (28lbs). He hasn't gone near beer and said I will never touch cocaine again. If you could please just pass this message on to Jason as a personal thank you for bringing out the 28-Day one. There is no way the other plans would have been enough. Lee is a very shy, skeptical person to say the least. If Jason wasn't doing his work, then how would people like my friend lee find a way, the right way! I'm sure he gets thank-you's everyday...But this one in particular is a special one. Lee knows I'm messaging Jason so if Jason wanted to use his name for anything he is welcome to...

Thank you Nina for taking the time out of your day to read this....

God bless you
Estella xxx

The reason this particular email stopped me in my tracks is this. Although I was aware of just how powerful this plan can be for weight loss and many *lifestyle related health conditions*, I didn't realize the impact it could also potentially have on other areas of someone's life, like addiction. This goes to illustrate that what we put into our bloodstream has a huge knock-on effect in many areas of our life, including the connections in our brain. *Super Juice Me!* is helping to change lives all over the world as we speak, and in many more ways than I ever imagined. Despite this *fact*, there are many people, who would rather, for reasons unknown to me, totally dismiss this concept or type of treatment as nothing more than *'quackery'*.

KNOCK KNOCK!
WHO'S THERE?
DOCTOR

There are many *'knockers'* of juicing in this world, especially, I am sad to say, within the medical profession. What I will say to critics of my approach is this: please read this book. Please read it with an open mind. Please see just how many people all over the world this is working for and, if you are brave enough, try it for yourself. There's an old saying, *'Don't knock it till you've tried it'*. I wish more people would just try it *before* they knock it – especially those in the medical industry, who have more influence over people's health than I. Please put aside your *'learned'* views on sugar, fibre and what constitute treatments for disease, and just try the programme yourself. Finish the full 28 days. Then, and only then, will you be in a truly informed position to knock it.

Lee's story is far from the only totally life-changing one. This book is littered with some truly phenomenal *Super Juice Me!* stories, all of which are there to inspire and give confidence to those embarking on the plan.

If you do have the courage of your convictions and are inspired to get *'Super Juiced'* yourself, please drop me a line. The more stories that come in, the more they will be forced to listen.

Good luck

May The Juice Be With You!

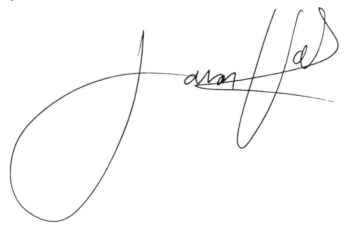

SUPER JUICE ME!

THE BIG JUICE EXPERIMENT

1

When I took eight people with 22 different diseases between them and put them on nothing but freshly extracted vegetable and fruit juices for 28 days, I must admit I expected some good results. But even I wasn't ready for just how utterly incredible the results would be.

If you have seen the documentary *Super Juice Me!*, you will already know what happened and be fully aware of what I am talking about. If you haven't watched the film, then make sure you do so before you embark on this 28-Day *Super Juice Me! Juice Plan*. Nothing, I believe, will inspire you more. Since the initial launch of the film in the Odeon Leicester Square in London's West End, over one million people have seen it and it's still very early days – it was only released a few months ago. *Super Juice Me!* is currently being shown on Virgin Atlantic flights across the world, and *Hello!* magazine are about to give the film free to all their readers after the editor watched the movie, loved it and felt it would make a difference!

The documentary came about simply because of what I had personally experienced on a juice-only diet and because of what I had been observing for years at my juice retreats. It also came about because of the tens of thousands of emails I received from people all over the world who had experienced enormous transformations in their health and weight due to following, in-particular, *7lbs in 7days Juice Master Diet*.

When I first started to receive these life-changing emails I might have, like most, dismissed them as purely anecdotal. However, when thousands upon thousands of emails come in all reporting exactly the same thing, it's time to sit up and pay attention.

With each email it became more and more apparent that seemingly most *lifestyle disease* would either improve or go away altogether if a person did two very simple things:

1. <u>Stop</u> the rubbish (pollution) coming into the body
2. <u>Start</u> putting in the right nutrition

Moreover, it soon became crystal clear that if a person went on an *exclusively* freshly extracted *raw* juice diet for a set period of time, the body would start to heal itself, almost regardless of how a person, or medics for that matter, named their particular disease.

Take my own case as an example. I was covered from head to foot in a skin disease called psoriasis; I couldn't even wear jeans without my skin cracking. I also had extremely severe asthma, eczema and hay fever. Although my diseases all had different names, they *all* healed, to a greater or lesser degree when I started to do these two simple things:

1. Stopped putting rubbish into my body
2. Started putting in the *right* nutrition

I am aware that this is far too simplistic for many, especially some in the medical profession, but why does it need to be complicated? All wild animals without exception consume *only* the food nature designed for them and in a *raw* and *live* state. At the same time, they do not suffer anywhere near the same level of disease that we humans do. In fact, the amount of disease in the wild pales into complete insignificance compared to what we humans experience. It is true that animals do indeed get things like arthritis, skin problems, diabetes, and so on, but the vast majority of those animals with these conditions are under human control. In other words, the second we control what animals as pets or in zoos eat, it all starts to go wrong!

I am not saying for one second that all disease can be 'cured' by simply jumping on the juice wagon for a set period of time, so please never misquote me for your headlines by saying such a thing. What I am saying is, when it comes to the vast majority of *lifestyle* diseases big health improvements can be made if a person does just those two things:

1. Removes the toxicity
2. Replaces the deficiencies

This is all that happened during the *Super Juice Me!* 28-Day experiment. I simply put all eight people, with 22 'different' diseases between them, on the *live* and *raw* juice diet. The diet was devised with just these two fundamental key healing principles in mind:

1. **The removal of *all* toxicity coming into the body**
2. **The replacement of any nutritional deficiencies.**

All 8 people were put on an exclusive, well thought-through, juice-only diet for 28 days. During that time they had no cooked, denatured or chemical-laden food or drink. All of the juices were freshly extracted and as such were *raw* and *live*. All eight people consumed only the juices I had devised for them, nothing else.

As part of the experiment, I also lived along side them, consuming only the juices they were having for the whole 28 days.

To make sure the 'Super Juicers' couldn't accuse me of not experiencing the same detox or withdrawal symptoms as they were, I effectively supersized myself before I 'Super Juiced' myself. For five weeks before the *Super Juice Me!* experiment, I ate and drank things I hadn't had for many years, and in large quantities. I soon found out that, while some people have great muscle memory, I have a very good 'fat memory'! I also didn't do any exercise, and managed to pile on 20lbs in just five weeks.

Yes, I ate a lot! I also felt like I'd just been run over by a truck and it was a reminder of how I used to feel every day. I wanted to experience the same withdrawal from white refined sugar, caffeine and refined fats as the people taking part in the experiment. I also wanted to see how easy or hard it actually was if you were coming off those drug-like foods and drinks. I had lived on nothing but juice for three whole months when

I first started juicing – over 15 years ago now – and I'd found that very difficult. At that time I didn't fully understand what I was doing and I was using 'diet mentality' (more about this in a later chapter), which makes it unnecessarily difficult. However, I wanted to see what happened this time with my far better understanding of nutrition and psychology.

I made sure that all the freshly extracted juices contained the right balance of nutrients to not only meet the Super Juicers' daily energy needs, but to also replace any nutritional deficiencies they may have been suffering from. If you are thinking 'juice diet equals carton orange and apple juice' for 28 days, you couldn't be further from what we were all actually having. The fresh juices from broccoli, cucumber, carrot, courgette, spinach, ginger, celery, apple, pineapple, kale, lemon, mint, to name but a few, all played a starring role during the *Super Juice Me!* experiment. As well as the juices, things like avocado or banana were blended with the juices a couple of times a day for added insoluble fibre and essential fats. Wheatgrass shots, hemp and spirulina were also added to the programme for extra iron and protein.

Now I don't want to spoil the film for you if you haven't yet seen it, but the whole point of this book is two-fold:

1. To illustrate how effective this plan can be for many health conditions.
2. To inspire you to take the *Super Juice Me! 28-Day Juice Challenge.*

To kick things off, here's an email that Dr Justine (the doctor who was involved in the documentary) received from one of the participants a couple of months after he had finished the *Super Juice Me! 28-Day Juice Challenge*:

Hi Justine,

Well, I am really well, so well that it's, well – quite hard to describe!

I spent almost three years being ill with lupus, bloated by steroids, overweight, depressed and suffering from the side effects of steroids and other drugs – but now, nothing but rude good health!

Since being back home, I have refurbished the front of the house, chain sawed trees and logs to fill our log store and done plenty of other active DIY and gardening. Yesterday, just as an example, I swapped the summer tyres and wheels on my Land Rover for the winter tyres and wheels that I have in store. Each wheel and tyre weighs around 30kg and I manhandled all eight of them with no problems at all.

On 15 September, I completed the Great North Run (the biggest half marathon in the world) – an achievement that I am really proud of and am still quite amazed that I could do it, particularly as in June this year I was finding it difficult to walk just 300 metres! I'll certainly be doing the Great North Run again next year!

The best part of getting my health back is the optimism and cheerfulness I feel as well as the fact that after a full day of physical work, I just feel pleasantly tired – not exhausted. Most of the things I have been doing recently, I just couldn't have even attempted a few months ago.

I am taking no drugs at all. My sleep apnoea and

snoring has gone and so has my CPAP machine – this means my wife and I now sleep together again every night, having previously spent over two years sleeping in separate bedrooms. The happiness this closeness has brought to both of us is worth everything!

I'm 67 years of age. In June being 67 felt dreadful – now being 67 feels no different to how I felt twenty years ago! The quality of life I've now got is great! I can never repay Jason and his team for this amazing change in my life.

Best Regards

Roger G

Here is a guy who could barely walk 300 metres before the *Super Juice Me! 28-Day Juice Experiment* who is now running the biggest half-marathon in the world (13.1 miles) just two months later! He and his wife couldn't sleep in the same room for over two years because he had to sleep with a CPAP (Continuous Positive Airway Pressure) machine, which uses mild air pressure to keep the airways open when someone with intermittent breathing is sleeping. These machines are noisy and an 'oxygen mask' has to be worn. They are also very expensive! Yet even before he had finished the *Super Juice Me!* experiment he had stopped using it. The impact this alone has had on his relationship is immeasurable. Roger told me personally that the programme not only saved his life but his marriage too. At the time of writing this book, over a year since the juice experiment, Roger is still *completely* drug and disease free. He has calculated that the *Super Juice Me!* experiment had saved the NHS (National Health Service in the UK) over £100,000 on him alone. No more sleep apnoea machine, no more drugs and no more need for the doc. This is quite an extraordinary turnaround in just 28 days on nothing but juice.

Another one of the participants, Sarah Crosby, sent me this email three months after the *Super Juice Me!* Big Juice experiment:

> On the Crohn's front – I'm still 100% medication free & I can't believe it. Well, I can, it makes perfect sense, but I'm just completely in awe of the entire process. Still healing to be done of course, that'll take some time but with the results I've had so far- incredible. I know it's easy to say, but I do feel like I have such a story to share with people. My Crohn's was so severe & debilitating, now I'm almost a PT- it shouldn't make sense but it does & I can't wait for the documentary so more people with IBD see it & realize that it's possible to control without a trailer full of medication.
>   Life changing!'
>
> **Sarah C**

Crohn's Disease can be one of the most incredibly debilitating conditions a person can suffer from, and Sarah Crosby had not had a single pain-free day for over year before she turned up to take part in the documentary. I won't spoil the film if you haven't seen it, but the improvements that every participant experienced by the time the 28 days were up were quite remarkable.

Since the launch of the film, thousands more have jumped on the *Super Juice Me! 28-Day Juice Challenge* and have experienced unbelievable results. I will share these throughout the book, as nothing will inspire more than hearing the stories of those it has worked for. Just the small colour section in the middle of this book would usually be all the inspiration a person needs to jump on board.

However, despite this truly breath-taking turnaround in Roger's health, as well as in others who took part in the film, and the quite extraordinary positive health changes in the thousands upon thousands more who have been 'Super Juiced' since then, many doctors, dieticians and the like have attacked the *Super Juice Me! 28-Day Challenge* as either, 'nutritionally unsound', 'unscientific' or 'dangerous'.

If we take Roger as an example here, we need to bear in mind that he had been on various concoctions of medical drugs for *years* on end and he was still very, *very* sick when he arrived for the juice experiment. The drugs he had been taking every single day for years did not make him well. He was also suffering from a multitude of adverse side effects from these drugs, side effects which were making him sicker, not better. This is why I find it somewhat ironic that certain people – not all, clearly – in the medical profession advise those with health challenges not to embark on the *Super Juice Me! 28-Day Challenge*, often claiming that it's dangerous! I can think of many things in life which are genuinely dangerous – sticking your head in a hot oven, heading to a war zone, hanging off a 100ft crane, to name a few – but living on freshly extracted fruit and vegetable juices and some extremely good nutritional supplements for 28 days is not one of them! Why do some in the medical profession feel that it's in some way better and *less dangerous* for a patient to continue eating and drinking rubbish while *adding* a plethora of medical drugs to their daily intake, than drinking freshly extracted juice for a month? If a person is overweight and sick with a lifestyle-related disease and the drugs aren't making them well, what harm could there be in at least trying this?

And that's the point really, harm. We need to always remember that, as far back as Hippocrates' time, the oath that medics once swore was:

FIRST DO NO HARM

It's an old oath, which seems to have been lost in some medical circles, and many think nothing of trying one drug after another to see if any of them make a difference. In *Super Juice Me!* I conducted a 'Big Juice Experiment', but it appears the pharmaceutical industry and medics have been conducting 'The Big Drug Experiment' on millions of people for many years. If this particular drug doesn't work, try that one. If that doesn't work, try this drug. And so it goes on and on, almost without regard to the potential adverse side effects or to addressing the *cause* of the problem, but simply trying drug after drug to treat the *symptoms*. We are only talking about the freshly extracted juices from the food nature designed for every cell in our body. Why is that deemed by many in the medical profession as 'dangerous' while drug therapy seemingly isn't?

You may deduce from what I'm saying that I am indeed anti-doctor and anti-pharmaceutical drugs. You may even, especially if you are a medic, think I am in the crackpot 'alternative' camp, where some believe that dissolving a sugar – sorry, *homeopathic* – pill under your tongue or hovering your hands over someone while they close their eyes can cure every disease on earth. This is not the case as I will fully explain in the 'GOLDFISH BOWL' chapter (page 57) and have already touched on in the prologue. I don't go around calling myself a 'healer', promising miracles with aid of the 'energy' I can transmit from my healing hands! It's those in that particular camp who, I believe, make it hard for professional medics to take any alternative therapy seriously. Unfortunately, they put us all in the same camp.

I wish to be crystal clear about this. Without the very *medical* asthma pump which I used to take many times a day, I believe I wouldn't be alive today. I am convinced of that. As I keep repeating throughout this book, so there is no chance of any confustion, I am not against *short-term* medical drug use; it is absolutely necessary at times. And to be honest, long-term medical drug use is also necessary in certain cases. What I am completely against is the over-prescribing of drugs and keeping people on them for life *unnecessarily*, simply for financial gain. I am also completely against the immediate dismissal by so many doctors of anything deemed 'alternative', even if it is based on good sound nutritional principles and, more importantly, is working!

For example, I would fully understand any medic, scientist or dietician attacking the juice experiment if the *Super Juice Me! Challenge* either had no effect on the people taking part or made them worse. But why would anyone attack something that had helped someone to turn their health around? Why would anyone, especially those who entered their profession with the sole aim of helping people in the area of health, not fully embrace a programme that enabled someone like Roger, for example, to remove *all* of his medical drugs plus a CPAP machine from his life? Why would anyone in the medical profession not at least look into any treatment which effectively gave a person their life back, where medical drugs had completely failed? How or why would medic look at something like Charlie Green's hand (see colour pages), let alone her extraordinary weight loss, and not embrace the method which completely cured it? How or why would any medic not at least look into it, even a little, rather than just dismissing it as 'non-medical quackery'?

A DOCTOR A DAY KEEPS THE APPLE AWAY

Many medics still scoff, often quite loudly and in my direction, at any type of nutritional therapy as a genuine treatment for disease. It all gets put into the alternative 'fruitcake' zone. Not once did any medical professional ask what I was eating and drinking when determining what treatment was needed for my severe psoriasis, eczema and asthma – not once. What I was putting into my body was completely irrelevant as far as they were concerned.

I even heard one extremely respected doctor say several times on BBC television and radio, no less, 'Diet has no effect on skin conditions'. I am not joking. The doctor said this on more than one occasion. My complaint to the BBC fell on deaf ears, as it so often does when it comes to this subject. If the World Health Organization acknowledges that between 70 and 85 per cent of all disease is caused by what we put into our mouths and by lack of physical movement, then why didn't anyone in the medical profession ask what I was eating and drinking before dishing out the drug pills or the 'burn your skin off' steroid creams for my skin condition? Why did my diet never *ever* come up in conversation with any doctor or dermatologist during the entire time I was being treated?

This honestly blows my mind. I don't understand how we managed to put a man on the moon in the 1960s, and yet in 2015 nutritional therapy still isn't seen as a credible treatment for disease when the wrong nutrition is *known* to be the cause of a great deal of it? How has this happened? If lifestyle diseases are just that, caused by *lifestyle*, then you don't need six years' worth of medical training or the brains of a NASA scientist to work out that a change in *lifestyle* is probably needed in order to reverse a *lifestyle* disease.

We are pretty much conditioned from birth to think 'doctor knows best' in every situation, even when it goes against our natural instinct and common sense. It is, I feel, extremely hard to argue that liver-toxic medical drugs, often with harmful side effects, are a better treatment for many lifestyle diseases than good solid nutrition and physical movement. It becomes even harder to argue when the overwhelming evidence suggests otherwise. That overwhelming evidence is coming in daily, and it's becoming more and more difficult for the medical industry to ignore it or dismiss it as 'purely anecdotal'. As I have said – and I feel the need to keep repeating it, for obvious reasons – I am not saying for one second that *Super Juice Me!* is a cure-all. I'm not saying it's a 'cure-anything', but unlike many medical drugs, it adheres to the old doctor's oath, 'First do no harm'. More importantly the *Super Juice Me!* programme is working on many levels for thousands of people all over the world. I believe it is working to such an extent that it would be almost criminal if the medical profession didn't look seriously at it.

As mentioned above, the aim of this book is not simply to lay out the full *Super Juice Me! 28-Day Challenge* – you can get that simply from a shopping list and a few pages – but to inspire you to actually do it! I don't know you, or your situation, but I do know that many people reading this book have suffered for years with either obesity or illness. You don't pick up a book of this nature if all is well in the health camp. I am also fully aware that many people reading this will already have tried a great deal of what the medical profession has to offer and, like Roger from the *Super Juice Me!* film, have had no success.

Whatever words I can try and muster in order to inspire you to start, I will. I am fully aware that my style of writing isn't for everyone. I use 20 words where two would have done very nicely, and I repeat the same points over and over again. I know this can be jarring at times, but please just ride with it; the prize at the end is beyond worth it. Just so you know, I repeat things not because I have I forgotten that I have already mentioned it, but to hammer home the same point in a slightly different way. It may be just one point put slightly differently which resonates with you personally and inspires you to go from *thinking* about doing this to *actually* doing it. Long before I found the juice, I studied addiction psychology and I learnt the power of repetition then. That's all advertisers do, repeat the same message over and over again until you finally act. This is why I make no apology for certain key points being repeated throughout this book. It is a form of conscious hypnosis, so please ride with it.

I also make no apology for the, let's say, colourful language I use at times or the many testimonials scattered within these pages. I have done all of this with just one purpose in mind: to get you to act! And when it comes to getting you to act, nothing I say can be anywhere as effective as the stories of real people who have had real results doing this plan. There is no question the film will go a long way in helping to inspire you to start. Since the film was launched, thousands more have done the *Super Juice Me! 28-Day Challenge*, often with truly remarkable results. The stories you are about to read are 100 per cent genuine and unsolicited; not one has been doctored or exaggerated in any way. When I was looking for stories and emails to give good examples of the success people have with the *Super Juice Me!* Challenge, it was almost impossible to choose. I have thousands to choose from! Please make a point of reading all of them, as they each tell their own story of what is possible.

I have also commented on each one. Many of the key points about sugar, for example, are to be found in those comments. I have made a point of doing it that way so that you read the letters, stories *and* comments after them. It's easy to just flick through a book, but to fully understand the potential power of what you are about to embark on and be more fired up than ever, it's imperative you read everything in the book. You should also make sure you don't lose momentum. Commit to reading at least four pages of this book every day, otherwise it will become yet another slightly read self-help book that you never acted on. It is called self-help because you have to help yourself. I cannot read the book or do the challenge for you, but I do know that if you commit to reading the book your chances of actually committing to do the programme go up exponentially.

Now, I've have had the privilege of receiving some incredible emails over the years from people who have read and completed my *7lbs in 7days Juice Master Diet*, but they are nothing in comparison to the emails which are filling my inbox everyday from people declaring…

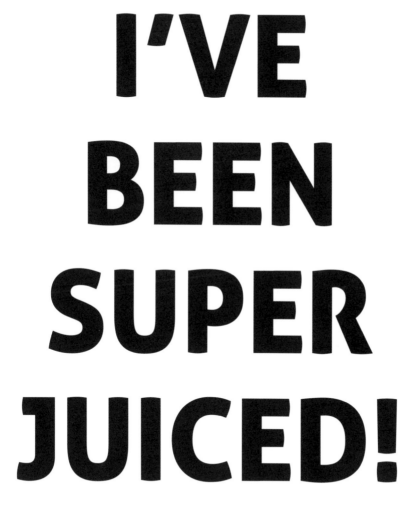

I'VE BEEN BEEN SUPER JUICED!

2

LOST 20LBS, ECZEMA ALMOST VANISHED AND FEEL ON TOP OF THE WORLD!

WOOHOOO I have just been super juiced. What an amazing journey. I began this journey to lose weight but also to regain control of my life.

I was 20kgs over weight, NEVER ate vegetables in fact I HATED vegetables (yet managed the drinks absolutely fine, in fact they were delicious), LOVED anything sweet, had really dry skin and was covered in eczema. I would coat myself in hydrocortisone most days so I didn't scratch myself to pieces. I now only have a **very, very small patch of eczema left** so hopefully by the end of next month it will be gone for good.

But best of all I have lost 9.1kgs!

I have lost:
7.5cm off my waist,
5.5cm off my hips,

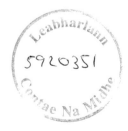

5cm off my left thigh,
6cm off my right thigh
2cm off both of my calves.

I feel on top of the world and can't wait to continue the next step and continue to lose the next 10.9kg in time for my wedding. The app was amazing but what really made me gain control of my life was the amazing book – Slim for Life. This opened my eyes and truly changed the way I look at food.

SUGAR, I was addicted to the stuff. Yesterday at morning tea there was chocolate and do you know what...it didn't interest me in the slightest. People who know me may have said pigs flew that day.

So Jason and Team *THANK YOU*. You have changed my life in more ways than you will ever know.

Lauren D

The weight and inch loss is quite dramatic here. Lauren dropped 20lbs in 28 days and an even more impressive 7.5 cm from her waist. Even more striking is the effect the programme has had on her eczema. She was covered in this skin condition and would coat herself in a topical corticosteroid daily to get some respite. After just 28 days she now has, 'only a very, very, small patch of eczema left'. This is why I got extremely frustrated when I heard that well-respected doctor on BBC Radio 2 say, 'Diet plays no part in skin conditions like psoriasis, eczema and acne'.

Once again I am not saying this is a cure for eczema – or anything else for that matter – but it clearly has had a major effect on this woman's skin, just as it had a monumental effect on my skin. So, for a doctor to dismiss diet altogether when it comes to possible causes and treatments for skin conditions is not only wrong but it also stops people from even trying a change in diet, just because the person with the white coat told them not to bother.

★   ★   ★

DROPPED 10LBS, CHOLESTEROL 5.6 TO 4.2, BMI 23.5 TO 20.2, 99% OF JOINT PAIN RECEDED

I can honestly say you haven't lived until you've been "Jason Vale'd".

I went on the 28-Day *Super Juice Me!* for health reasons. In my vanity, I assumed I didn't need to shift any weight, well maybe a couple of pounds.

My aim was to get rid of my insomnia (I haven't slept through the night in 9 years), get rid of my IBS and ease the aches and pains in my bones and joints caused by Chemo and Radiotherapy. After the first few days I started to sleep through the night and wake without feeling dizzy or having a nagging headache, IBS disappeared after 10 days and 99 per cent of bone and joint pains have receded. I never felt hungry! Cravings went after the first couple of days. My vitals are: cholesterol from 5.6 down to 4.2; BMI from 23.5 down to 20.2 and lost 10lbs/4.5 kilos; blood pressure/sugars have always been low, so no change there. All I can say is don't knock it until you try it, then there is no going back. I will be J-J-M-ing from now on. That's two juices/smoothies and one meal per day.

Sara B

Where do we start? Dropped 10lbs, IBS gone after just ten days, never felt hungry, 99 per cent of joint and bone pain gone, BMI down from 23.5 to 20.2, and reduced cholesterol. This, remember, all happened in just 28 days! This is why this must be looked at seriously by the medical profession as a genuine form of treatment for many 'different' diseases. I know some people who have tried every medical drug on earth for IBS and have never had any real respite. Yet here's someone who after just ten days was completely symptom free. Ninety-nine per cent of her joint pain has also gone, without any drug-based anti-inflammatories. As I will point out later, but worth mentioning here, some form of inflammation causes the vast majority of lifestyle disease and fruits and vegetables are natural anti-inflammatories. This is why, when you remove *all* the toxic, inflammatory foods and drinks for 28 days and replace them with *only* natural anti-inflammatory juices, many lifestyle diseases begin to improve so dramatically. You will also notice that this woman has also vowed to carry on J-J-M-ing (Juice-Juice-Meal) and says 'there's no going back'. You'll notice she hasn't decided to go back to her old ways at the end of the programme. She feels so good she doesn't want to lose that feeling and go back. And isn't that the whole point? Not only to get the results of the 28-Day juice challenge, but ultimately to have life-long change on the back of it.

★   ★   ★

DROPPED 28LBS IN 28 DAYS!

Jason Vale is a God-send!! I watched the movie twice so far and I suspect I'll watch it again sometime. I vigorously jumped on the *28-Day Super Juice Me!* programme after watching the movie at the beginning of May, and I completed it yesterday – I feel great, woo hoo!! I've lost almost 2 stones (28lbs), and the easiest way to describe how I feel is balanced! No complaints whatsoever!! I'm now embarking on Jason's recommendation of J-J-M and I'm still excited about it all! I wasn't ill, but my health has improved, my waistline is cinched and my energy levels have gone way up! Thank you Jason Vale Juice Master, I am now a daily juicer!!

Rubee R

If you want to do this programme for weight loss, I can honestly say I don't know of anything else that is more effective in this area than a juice-only programme. She is far from the only person who has dropped 28lbs in just 28 days;

this is just one out of hundreds of stories to illustrate what many are experiencing. If someone has a lot of weight to lose, then they will drop about 1lb a day; many lose a great deal more, as you'll see in the next letter…

★   ★   ★

BLOOD PRESSURE REDUCED, LYMPHOEDEMA HALVED IN SIZE, WEIGHT LOSS: 37LBS FOR HER AND 33LBS FOR HIM

Two years ago I discovered I had breast cancer and a rare skin and muscle disease called dermatomyositis. I am still recovering from both. However, I have put on a massive amount of weight, with not being able to move very much and all medication, steroids, etc. 4 weeks ago My partner, Barry, and I started *Super Juice Me!* 28lbs in 28 days….I can't believe it. Barry lost 37lbs and I lost 33lbs. It's amazing, my blood pressure has went from very high to 115/75 and my cholesterol is now 4. I had very, very bad water retention in my legs and feet and lymphedema in my left arm, which has now halved in size. Thank you so much I can't tell you how much this has helped me.

Angie H

This lady dropped 33lbs and her husband a whopping 37lbs in just 28 days. The average weight loss a person will experience on a conventional diet is 2lb a week. This means it would have taken the husband almost 20 weeks to achieve the same results as just four weeks on the *Super Juice Me!* plan. Angie herself not only lost 33lbs but also lowered her blood pressure, her cholesterol, and her lymphoedema has halved.

★   ★   ★

STOPPED TAKING METFORMIN!
SUGAR LEVELS NORMAL
WEIGHT LOSS: 15LBS

Just finished day 28...and starting another 28 days! Feeling so amazing!

I really did enjoy it. My sugar levels are normal, and I've stopped taking Metformin (yeah!). I have more energy then I've had in years! I've started cycling in spite of fibromyalgia, as my muscles and joints don't hurt, so that has increased my activity levels...and I've lost 15lbs in the process!

I FEEL AMAZING!!

Sheila B

Metformin is an anti-diabetic drug which works by suppressing glucose production by the liver. One of the arguments many medics and dieticians use against the *Super Juice Me!* programme is 'sugar'. They claim, wrongly, that all sugars are the same and anyone with diabetes shouldn't juice but always eat whole, or it will cause further blood-sugar issues and exacerbate their type 2 diabetes.

Here is a lady who was on an anti-diabetic drug and stopped taking it during a month of drinking nothing but freshly extracted juices. According to current medical and dietetic thinking this shouldn't be possible because of all the sugar. But not all sugars are built the same (see Q&A, page 341), and this woman is far from the first to regulate her blood sugars on the *Super Juice Me!* programme. While we were filming *Super Juice Me!*, a man whose normal seven-day juice detox at the retreat coincided with the last week of the *Super Juice Me!* experiment was extremely worried because of his diabetes about having juice only. I told him to keep a check on his blood sugar and to come to me immediately if anything was wrong. On day 5 he came up to me and said he didn't understand what was happening. He had reduced his insulin intake by 75 per cent. Let me repeat that, because it goes totally against what everyone is being told by the 'all sugars are the same brigade': **in just five short days he had reduced his insulin intake by 75 PER CENT**.

I totally agree that shop-bought cooked or pasteurized juice is not good for diabetics, but shop-bought juice and the freshly extracted variety you will be consuming when Super Juicing yourself on this plan are worlds apart on every level. Clearly, if you are diabetic you must consult your doctor first before doing this plan. However, if you do consult your doctor please do your best to explain you'll be consuming freshly extracted vegetable and fruit juices with blended avocado, and not pasteurized apple juice from a carton!

Not only did this woman regulate her blood sugars and remove her need for diabetic medicine but she's even started cycling in spite of her fibromyalgia, as her muscles and joints no longer hurt. She's also dropped 15lbs into the bargain and feels amazing. Not bad for just 28 days!

★   ★   ★

ULCERATIVE COLITIS UNDER CONTROL FOR FIRST TIME IN 2 YEARS WEIGHT LOSS: 26LBS

I'VE BEEN SUPER JUICED! I've just completed the 28-Day *Super Juice Me!* I've lost 26 pounds, I feel fab and my colitis is under control for the first time in 2 years! Thank you, thank you, thank you Jason and team, I don't think I could have done it without the app. I've had ulcerative colitis for 2 years, I'd just finished 6 months of steroids and my symptoms started again within a week! I was started on chemotherapy drugs!! I was feeling lower than low and just thought "that's it!" I bought the app for my iPad that day, ordered my fruits and veg and just did it. The first 4 days were hard, massive headache from tea withdrawal, but on day 5 I had no headache, my

PR bleeding had stopped and I actually caught myself singing and dancing whilst prepping the veggies! I HAD to carry on. The weight loss is an amazing bonus, 24 inches smaller all over, my clothes don't fit me now and I've got loads of energy. The app really helped, it was like having Jason there to talk me through it (a book is easy to ignore). I'm going to carry on with the juicing and have one evening meal (low H.I.). The most surprising thing is that I haven't craved chocolate or crisps, both of which I was having nearly every night. My first meal will be stir fried broccoli, mushroom and garlic, nom nom nom

Emily C

The main thing I wish to point out here is that this woman had been on steroid treatment for six whole months, and her symptoms started again within one week of ending the steroids. Not only that, but the medical profession put her on chemotherapy drugs! Yet within just five days on the *Super Juice Me!* plan her bleeding had stopped. She has managed to get her ulcerative colitis fully under control for the first time in over two years. On top of that, she dropped 26lbs and 24 inches off her body. Please also observe that her cravings for chocolate and crisps (that's potato chips for my American friends) also went, and her first meal – out of genuine choice – was a healthy one. Not only does the *Super Juice Me!* plan potentially have the power to help various lifestyle diseases, but it can also 'reset' the mind and remove the desire for junk food.

★   ★   ★

RESTING HEART RATE DROPPED FORM 59PBM TO 42BPM REDUCED SYMPTOMS OF FIBROMYALIGIA

MY WIFE IS A 28-DAY SUPER JUICER...

After 28 days of juicing, Julie has gone from strength to strength on Jason Vale's *28-Day Super Juice Me* plan.

Julie has lost close to a stone in weight (14lbs), dropped her resting heart rate to 42 from 59bpm, massively reduced her symptoms of fibromyalgia, lost all sugar cravings, stopped all aches in her knees and improved in many other ways both physically and mentally. Julie has also been able to train hard with Luke in preparation for them to do a 100 mile section of the Camino de Santiago later this year with me. Julie is making this just the start of re-balancing her lifestyle – mind, body and soul and will continue indefinitely...eating highly nutritious, organic veggie and fruit juices.

I am proud to see that Julie has turned a BIG corner in her road back to fitness and health. The difference in her is just amazing and all through relatively small changes.

Live Your Life...Love Your Life

Tim G

Once again here's someone with fibromyalgia who has seen massive improvements in her condition on the programme. She has also dropped a stone (14lbs) in weight and her sugar cravings are gone! What I love is how her husband said, 'The difference in her is just amazing and all through relatively small changes'. Although the *Super Juice Me!* plan appears to be one of massive change, it is relatively small considering what has been achieved. I agree that *Super Juice Me!* does seem quite drastic on the surface, but it's nowhere near as drastic as many of the medical drugs which are given out left right and centre, often unnecessarily and often with quite debilitating side-effects.

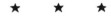

BEEN SUPER JUICED AND GOING ON TO JUICE FOR 56DAYS! WEIGHT LOSS: 3 STONE (42LBS)

Just completed the 28-Day Plan and I dropped from 21 stone (294lbs) to 18 stone (252lbs) on day 26! I decided I am not stopping here so I stopped watching the day 26 video and moved on! Here I am on day 28 and tomorrow is day 29 of 56! My goal is to drop from 18 stone (252lbs) now to 14 stone! (196lbs) I know I can do it!!

Super Juice Me! Is a great plan, my journey has been fantastic and the coaching videos are spot-on, talking about how some people are 'dementors' on week 1. In particular the week 3 video about being lonely was spot on as was week 4 about the high of completing my 28 days. My weight loss was great, I tried to keep to the plan as much as I could and as much at my pocket would allow me too. But there were days when I improvised because I ran out of certain ingredients. But it was very easy, through the whole journey. People say I should work for Juice Master because everything I have learned I have passed on to other people and inspired so many of my family and friends, who are all now going to do the plan. My sister is now about to start the 28 day plan which hopefully will inspire my mum to do it properly, but I believe the only way is to send her to the Juicy Oasis. I am currently saving the money up to get her out there for the 28 day plan because I believe she needs to be in this environment to kick start this journey for her.

Mitesh J

This guy has dropped 42lbs in just 28 days! Some medics say it's not good to lose this much weight so quickly, and then go on to massively contradict themselves by putting obese people in for bariatric surgery. This is where they turn the stomach from the size of a large fist to the size of a thumb. After surgery, patients often lose tremendous amounts of weight extremely quickly and some lose their appetite altogether and have to force themselves to eat for fear of malnutrition. All that the *Super Juice Me!* plan has done is to enable this person to drop a huge amount of weight in a very small space of time in an extremely healthy and risk-free way. Bariatric surgery has huge risks attached and isn't as successful as they make out. What is 'success' after all? Many who have this type of surgery go into deep depression and require massive amounts of aftercare. The success of *Super Juice Me!* has also spurred him on to continue until he hits a very healthy 196lbs. That would be over 100lbs weight loss, using only what nature has to offer. No pills, no surgery!

★   ★   ★

DROPPED 28LBS / 5 INCHES OF MY WAIST / 2 DRESS SIZES/ DEPRESSION LIFTED/ IBS GONE

Here's my summary of being 'Superjuiced'. I cannot say for sure exactly what it was that convinced me to do this but it was on the day of the premiere in London. I was (as we all are) blown away by Jason's passion in the film and everybody's stories, their honestly, humility and commitment. I came away wishing that I could get all my friends who suffer to just try this out and made it a mission to spread the word ... but after the film I found myself very contemplative. I searched out a juice bar (the times I've gone straight to a pub with the new pack of cigarettes and parked myself for a session!) and sat and thought about all the tests and investigations I'd had, all the pills I'd been offered, all the pain I've been in, and how rubbish I'd felt for years and that only since juicing I had begun to improve my health and change my life – why not try this, why not kick myself once and for all firmly up my large butt into a new me! So I did and to my surprise – I bl***y did it! I have to admit, I did struggle occasionally, but never challenged about food, just tiredness at night at times but that could've been due to the amount of blinking stuff I've been doing! **It's like someone had literally plugged me in.** This stuff is nectar. My 5 year old says, "Mummy's having her petrol again, she'll be flying soon," and giggles! I can't fault the whole thing really and cannot advocate it enough. Any tough times I just tried to interpret as cleansing and cathartic. If you can exercise, it definitely helps. It gives you energy and is so cleansing. I turned to water often, and Pukka's Three Mint Tea is my new comfort blanket. The App is superb. Jason's videos hit all the right spots, totally supportive. I leapt and jumped and screamed and danced and cried and sang and twisted and sprung about in celebration. **Nothing short of the birth of my child has made me feel this good!** I am beginning to run – something I've always wanted to do and was only a dream to me – I was struggling to get to the top of my stairs. My joints were all in a mess (I have the beginnings of rheumatoid arthritis). I'm 45, but after getting out of bed in the mornings I was looking more like 85. I now jump out of bed and skip to the bathroom. My IBS pain/symptoms have subsided, juicing just stops it! This is heaven as it has controlled me for some time. **I'm supposed to be taking beta-blockers but I'm not and my symptoms have all gone, just gone – just like** that!!!!! **But best of all is the change in my mind set.** Depression has literally controlled the past few years of my life, I've been a prisoner to it – I've felt incapable of making a effort to make the drastic changes to my life that I desperately need to do in order to have a future. I didn't believe in me or any part of me...until now! **This is it...it's only the beginning but I really believe if I can keep my body this clean that my mind will stay strong and that I can actually do ANYTHING! I've lost nearly 2 stone. I've lost 5, yes 5, inches off my waist, 2in off my bust and my hips. I've dropped 2 sizes** and I've got into a dress that I couldn't get over my shoulders when it was given to me by a friend a few years ago! I'm blown away, just blown away. **I've cried tears of joy to feel so alive in a way I could only have dreamed of not so long ago.** Thank you, Jason and team, for giving me the tools to get my life back! Thank you all for this fantastic supportive page. Superjuicing is not for everyone...don't enter into it lightly, but, then again as Jason says, no one questions binge junk eating. Juicing is nectar, just nectar! Sorry I've gone on – I just can't express my joy without all this! I wish you all even a small measure of how I feel. I for one will continue to share the word.

Marie D

It's emails like the above which make me question why anyone in the medical or dietetic profession would ever knock this plan. Marie would struggle getting out of bed because of the beginnings of rheumatoid arthritis but now she jumps out of bed pain free. Her depression has lifted, she's dropped

28lbs, her IBS has gone and she says, 'Nothing short of the birth of my child has made me feel this good!' Why, with such incredible results, would anyone – let alone someone who is in their profession to help people – discourage anyone suffering with ill health or overweight from getting Super Juiced? Why are we still so logged into the 'pill for every ill' or 'cut them open' approach, often as a first point of call? Why are we in the position where so many people in the medical profession refuse to accept juice therapy as a credible way of treating certain conditions? When you read letters like the above, you do question what is happening in today's apparently modern, advanced and cutting-edge 'medical world'.

★   ★   ★

THIS MAY JUST BE THE BEST SOLUTION TO HEALTH PROBLEMS YET! PAIN AND 21LBS GONE!

I'VE BEEN SUPER JUICED!

Here are the results of my 28-day juice journey – **Lost 21lbs** (1.5 Stone)

I was injured in Afghanistan in 2009 and started dipping myself into a downward spiral when it came to my health and diet. I was always overeating; sometimes until I felt so full I could pop. I drank around 2-3 cans of Monster everyday and nothing else but can upon can of Coke. From 11st 4lb, rising rapidly to 15st 12lb, I was in need of serious help.

Not only was I gaining weight, my injuries from Afghanistan became painful, hurting everyday causing my mental health to deteriorate even further (I already suffering with PTSD). I was inspired by a friend that had recently done the 28-Day *superjuiceme* with fabulous results and I thought then that I need to – no, not need, I had to – do this for the sake of my health and well-being. I juiced and juiced, following the iPad app, and feeling the effects within days, I began to see my energy return, I started to feel amazing! The pain from my injuries began to lessen, the puffy sluggish feel began to vanish and I quickly realised that this is the plan that would change my life, this is going to be the new me. 28 days on and I feel absolutely fantastic, This may just be the best solution to health problems yet! I am going to be continuing to juice as part of my diet for the foreseeable future, mixing with a much better and healthy lifestyle. Jason, you are a truly remarkable man, and I would jump at the chance to attend your Juicy Oasis, and hopefully in the future I will be able to!

Thank you so much.

★   ★   ★

LOST ALL MY CELLULITE!

My name's Anne-Marie and I've been Super Juiced! Day 29 and I feel great. I didn't do this for weight loss and I don't have any diseases (that I know about!). I have participated in Jason Vale Juice Master's juice and I'm definitely a convert. I love juice. It's awesome. Anyway, after watching Jason's documentary, I got inspired and I mostly just wanted to see what would happen if I did this for 28 days, and also if I could do this for 28 days! It turns out I lost 3.5kg, 5cm from my waist, 5.5cm from my hips and 5cm from my thighs. This is HUGE for me because I am petite (152cm). None of my pants fit me now (which is kind of annoying and exciting at the same time). I really didn't think I had that much to lose. The upside is now all my backpacking weight from last year is gone. Yay! Anyway, the BEST thing that happened was I lost pretty much all of my cellulite. This isn't something I was expecting but you can imagine my surprise when I looked in the mirror and noticed it was pretty much gone. Nothing has ever come close to juicing for removing cellulite (for me). If you're currently participating in *Super Juice Me!* good luck and keep going! The results are worth it.

Anne-Marie D

The emails and results I receive daily from people who have been, 'Super Juiced' could fill several books in themselves. They are all as breath-taking, powerful and inspirational as each other. For many, reading these alone is all they will need to make the decision to start. In fact, the chances are

– especially if you've already taken a glance at the colour pages in the centre of the book, which show a few of the results – you'll be itching to get cracking.

However, it is extremely important that you are fully armed on every level before you start, and it's equally vital you have a full understanding of *why* this programme is working for so many people and for many apparently different diseases. I say, 'apparently different' diseases because over the past 15 years of doing this and after receiving thousands upon thousands of life-changing emails like the ones you've read just now, I do not believe there are in fact thousands of different diseases, but, rather, one main disease with various symptoms. These very different symptoms then get named as specific diseases in their own right and give the impression that we are subject to thousands of different diseases. We then treat each and every disease in isolation, believing it to be unique. This what drives BIG PHARMA to produce 'a pill for every ill and an ill for every pill', without anyone seemingly questioning if that's the best or even correct approach. I believe we have been going at it the wrong way for many years, and, specifically when it comes to the vast majority of lifestyle diseases, there aren't thousands of them with thousands of different solutions, but rather just …

ONE

DISEASE

WITH

ONE

SOLUTION

3

When I removed the majority of the rubbish from my diet, stopped my 40-60-a-day cigarette addiction, removed my heavy alcohol consumption and started adding freshly extracted juices, *every single aspect* of my mental and physical health started to improve.

The severe asthma I had had from the age of eight started to get better, and within a very short space of time I noticed I didn't need to use my asthma spray anywhere near as much. The chronic psoriasis which had covered my body from head to toe and plagued my life since I was 16 slowly began to get better. The eczema which had covered the backs of both of my knees and would crack each morning also started to vanish. The bloating and stomach cramps I suffered on a weekly basis started to become a rarity instead of the norm. And the excess weight which I had been carrying around with me for years just started to drop off.

As I continued, things improved by the week, if not by the day. In a very short space of time I had no need at all for my asthma spray, none at all. My asthma had genuinely vanished. This debilitating breathing condition, which prevented me doing what I loved most in the world, playing football, had somehow, out of nowhere, simply gone! No more need for the asthma spray drug and no further need to opt out of sports.

While that was happening, I slowly noticed large areas of skin becoming clear. My psoriasis hadn't gone completely, but I could see clear normal skin developing in areas where the psoriasis had been. I noticed I was no longer lethargic, and my thinking was clearer and sharper. I felt more positive, generally less stressed and more calm and happy. I am aware that these 'general wellness feelings' are subjective and 'unscientific'. However, the eczema vanishing, the psoriasis improving and the excess weight disappearing before my eyes are all very real and non-subjective. I wasn't taking specific juices to treat any specific conditions; I simply cut out the dead rubbish and started to pour in raw live nutrition in the form of freshly extracted vegetable juices. Because I felt so much better and had an enormous amount of energy I also started to exercise on a regular basis, not because I felt I had to but because I wanted to.

THE LIGHT BULB MOMENT

Since those early days of diet change I have learnt a great deal more about nutrition, health and disease. I have learnt what I needed to *add* to the juices in order to get rid of my psoriasis completely. (I cannot even begin to describe the feeling of being able to wear short-sleeve tee shirts and shorts in the summer.) I have also learnt that there are many contributing factors that make up disease. I have also discovered that the more I studied this subject the *less* I knew. No you haven't misread. The more I studied the less I really knew. Anyone who has studied this subject should also testify to that too. Nutrition and disease are like a black hole which you never ever get to the bottom of – if you go about it the conventional way, that is. It wasn't until I had a 'light-bulb' moment, that things became stupidly clear. In fact, it became so clear I was kicking myself I hadn't seen it before. The light-bulb moment is my 'One Disease – One Solution' hypothesis.

It came about after years of reading literally thousands of letters from people who had read the books and adopted a similar lifestyle to mine. In particular, letters from people who had done my *7lbs in 7days Juice Master Diet*. People who had only set out to lose a bit of weight to fit into 'that dress' or their skinny jeans had found the most wonderful side effects of the juice-only programme. It is not an exaggeration to say that almost every common lifestyle ailment and disease has been mentioned over the years in relation to the seven-day juice diet. People started to notice that not only was the weight dropping off – an absolute given on the plan – but ailments they had suffered from for years were improving… rapidly!

THE BODY WANTS TO HEAL ITSELF
…IF IT IS GIVEN THE CHANCE TO

Arthritis, IBS, migraines, skin problems, bloating, constipation, high cholesterol, asthma, gout, type 2 diabetes – the list just went on and on. And because the vast majority of people who did the programme changed a great deal of their diet and went on to make juicing part of their *daily* life, the number of ailments which appeared to be treated positively kept going up and up the longer someone continued with natural juice therapy.

The letters and emails were all from people I hadn't had a chance to see on a one-to-one basis. They were simply people who had read the book, stopped chucking heavily processed rubbish into their system and started to pour in the freshly extracted juice contained in nature's finest fuel.

On our juice retreats in Turkey and at Juicy Oasis in Portugal (where the film *Super Juice Me!* was filmed) I have witnessed with my own eyes the incredible healing power of the body. One woman at on the seven-day Turkish retreat had Crohn's Disease all of her life. She said there hadn't been a day she hadn't suffered the incredible discomfort from this debilitating disease. Just one week on fresh juices, no rubbish, some sunshine, no TV and a positive atmosphere and she was free from ALL symptoms for the first time in her adult life. Just seven days. Another lady came with severe arthritis, to the point where walking was incredibly difficult. Within one week she climbed a mini mountain (now called Monica's Mountain – hello Monica!). We have thousands of these stories, not just one or two. Thousands of *genuine* stories from regular people who desperately wanted some respite from their disease and got it from changing their diet and pouring some freshly extracted vegetable based juices into their system.

The one thing they all have in common is that they stopped polluting the system, added the right fuel and started to move their bodies.

YOU CANNOT HEAL SELECTIVELY

What the retreats, the letters and emails over the years and my own health experience and observations have made clear is this:

It doesn't matter what you name the lifestyle disease, they are all essentially part of the same one disease

It was Charlotte Gerson, daughter of the great juicing and health pioneer Max Gerson and founder of the Gerson therapy, speaking on the ground-breaking documentary *Food Matters*, who said, 'You cannot heal selectively. You cannot treat one disease and leave two untreated.' The whole body wants to heal. It will not treat one ailment and leave the rest untreated.

The body is at DIS-EASE. It is screaming to the person to stop the pollution, add the right fuel and clean the body so it can heal itself. Survival is number one as far as the body is concerned and it will do anything to keep you alive. Health comes second. The human body has a natural, powerful filtration system, designed to use what it can from whatever fuel enters the system and filter out the toxins.

The very same filter system kept me alive for years, despite my very excessive smoking, drinking and junk-food eating way of life. I was smoking two to three packets of cigarettes a day and drinking my own body-weight in alcohol, and I did this for years! It just shows the body is very good at doing whatever is needed to make sure it survives. The body did whatever it needed to do to gain whatever usable fuel it could from the crap I threw in. It did everything within its power to constantly filter the pollution which was flowing throughout my bloodstream and lungs.

But it can only do so much. It can only realistically deal with just so much crap every day. Pretty soon the pollution starts to take its toll. Pretty soon you get muzzy headed, lethargic, overweight, bloated. Years of polluting the system soon manifest itself in what we think of as *different* diseases. Asthma, eczema, psoriasis, IBS, migraines, depression, hay fever, diabetes, angina, obesity, endometriosis, gout, osteoporosis, etc. start to appear in our lives. And what have we been totally conditioned to do when this happens? Yes, we nip straight to our doctor and ask him or her to prescribe the best available drug to treat the *symptoms* of *that* particular disease.

A pill for every ill & an ill for every pill

We have been totally brainwashed to treat the symptoms and not even to consider what the cause may be. The cause, as you may already be gathering, is the same for the vast majority of people when it comes to the most common ailments and diseases: pollution entering the bloodstream on a daily and consistent basis, the over-burdening of the digestive system, and the lack of physical movement. The treatment, therefore, is to stop the pollution, feed the body the correct fuel it ultimately requires for optimum health, and help the lymphatic system (our internal filter system) do its job by doing some physical exercise.

MEDICAL VS ALTERNATIVE

Now, before I continue, I wish to make something very clear. I am talking about the vast majority of common ailments and diseases. I am *not* talking about *all* diseases. There are of course diseases, such as Type 1 Diabetes, which some people are born with, which absolutely require medical intervention and to which the 'One Disease – One Solution' hypothesis doesn't necessarily apply. This is one of the many reasons I am not against all medical drugs or medical approaches.

THE WARNING SIGNALS

We need to understand that the vast majority of disease doesn't just happen. You don't just wake up one day with a chronic disease. It can feel that way for sure, but it usually takes many, many years for that ailment or disease to manifest itself to the chronic stage. Cancer, for example, usually takes an average of 20 years to manifest itself.

If you are going to take full charge of your own health and that of the people you love the most, you need to start realizing that the body constantly sends you messages. It is often screaming for you to do something before things get to a stage at which it can't do anything about it. Unfortunately we are so conditioned to treat the symptoms of disease, even in its early stage, that we miss these vital signs. If we have a headache it appears most of us think we are low on aspirin, or if we get indigestion we are low on Rennie! We have been totally conditioned to treat our ills with pills, whilst ignoring the signals. It's like driving along in your car and the red warning light comes on telling you you're low on oil. But instead of taking the effort to stop the car and top up on oil, you rip out the red warning light instead!

Just because you can't see the problem doesn't mean it has gone away

Just because you take a drug to treat the *symptoms* of a disease and the symptoms of that condition subside for that moment, it doesn't mean the drug has solved or cured the problem.

For example, if I had a leaking roof and water was getting onto the ceiling tiles of the suspended ceiling below I wouldn't just replace the tiles, I would mend the roof. Unfortunately, so much of conventional medicine is based on the principle of replacing the ceiling tiles and ignoring the roof. If you ignore the roof, the hole in the roof will naturally get worse. The worse it gets, the more rain it lets in. The more rain it lets in, the larger the area of ceiling tiles that gets damaged. Now, who in their right mind would keep replacing more and more of the ceiling tiles without ever fixing the roof? Who in their right mind, when they replaced the ceiling tiles and all looked fine and dandy, would actually believe the situation has been even remotely solved. Ignore the roof and the ultimate cost to the house is potentially horrific, and in some cases irreversible. If we cover up the early warning signals when it comes to our health the ultimate price is one which money often can't fix.

When I had psoriasis every single person I saw in the medical profession was hell-bent on finding some kind of medical cream to put on my skin to treat the symptoms. They said there was no cure, so therefore they could only look at treating the symptoms. My body was screaming at me to clean my internal environment and supply the key nutrients so it could heal itself. I never once listened to the signs, even when they first started. I continued to pollute the system not only with the wrong foods, drinks, cigarettes and lack of exercise, but also with the drugs I was putting on my skin and into my body to treat the 'various' diseases I was suffering from.

The drugs themselves are poisons and add to the overall pollution. The side effects of the drugs cause further problems within the body, often causing a 'need' for more drugs to help treat those symptoms. And the disease–drug merry-go-round continues. A drug used to treat muscle pain could potentially cause kidney problems. But don't worry. There is another drug on hand that you can take for your new-found kidney problem. This drug may well have other side effects, such as breathing difficulties. However, once again don't despair. There is another prescription on hand for that, and so the pharma-side effect-pharma loop continues.

When I had my first asthma attack at the age of eight, both my mother and I thought I was going die. *IT WAS A WARNING!* My body was screaming at me, warning me there was something very, very wrong. When scabs appeared on the back of my knees and elbows, *IT WAS A WARNING!* The body was telling me something was up. When red patches started to appear and spread like wildfire all over my body, **IT WAS A WARNING!** When I started to develop breasts like a woman and wobble rather than move, IT WAS A WARNING! When I suffered from the world's worst migraines and had to shut the world out, IT WAS A WARNING! When I felt like crap, groggy and lethargic all the time, IT WAS A WARNING! But instead of asking myself what on earth was causing these problems, I simply popped pills, pumped on my asthma spray 14 times every day, and covered my body in drug cream. Why? Because, like almost all of us, I had been conditioned to think this way. It is only once something is pointed out that we have the opportunity to stand back, see how mad the whole approach is and seek a way to fix the roof.

I have taken just one medical drug in 10 years; it was for a back spasm, a pain which, unless you have experienced it, is almost impossible to comprehend. Medical intervention is often the only approach for pain relief and it's where medical professionals are quite brilliant. However, other than that one time, not a single medical pill or cream has gone in or on me for over 10 years now, and I have genuinely never felt or looked better. I can breathe without drugs, I have clear skin, I'm no longer fat and I feel mentally as sharp as a tack. I have cleared out the rubbish and provided the body with what it requires to heal and for *optimum* health. Remove the toxicity and replace the deficiencies and, in most cases, everything gets better.

WHAT A DIAMOND

One of my biggest mentors, Harvey Diamond (author of the Fit For Life series of books) summed it up in a reply to one of my emails, asking what he thought of my 'One Disease – One Solution' hypothesis:

Hi Jason

Very glad to hear that your approach is in the vein of "One Disease – One Solution", which for most people is beyond their comprehension. The medical community relies upon us believing that there are literally thousands of different possible ailments of the body and they alone know how to navigate through the confusion and complexity of them all and prescribe just the right drug to combat the particular ailment. I will readily admit that it is a difficult concept to accept by people who have been conditioned all their lives to believe otherwise, but in actual fact almost all so-called diseases have a similar cause, differentiated only by where in the body they occur. And, most encouraging of all is the fact that, once again despite the efforts to convince us otherwise, the remedy for all of these alleged ailments all come down to the utilization of a few basic, well proven and time tested principles; mainly a highly nutritious diet consisting primarily of living, uncooked food, support of the body's cleansing and healing mechanism (the Lymph System), regular exercise, and the avoidance of drugs. And so the medical community has spent the last 200 years or so trying to blame every ailment of the human body, which they do not understand and cannot explain, on mysterious, unseen forces that have as their only purpose the disease, ill health and destruction of human beings. In the vast majority of cases, the only connection that ill health has to unseen causes is the one medical doctors have made up for the purpose of deflecting attention away from the fact that they are ignorant of the true cause.

Harvey

Fit For Life was one of the first books I ever read on the subject of nutrition and it had a profound impact on my life. Harvey had been in the Vietnam war and was exposed to Agent Orange. When diagnosed with the 'no-known-cure' condition that destroys the muscles, he was told to prepare to die. Over 30 years later, and one of the very few remaining survivors with this debilitating condition, he credits his survival to maintaining a healthy and fluid lymph system. In other words, he was keeping the system free of toxicity whilst feeding it the finest nutrients.

'A POORLY FUNCTIONING IMMUNE SYSTEM THAT CAN'T FEND OFF TOXINS IS GUARANTEED TO CAUSE DISEASE ... ONLY A STRONG HEALTHY IMMUNE SYSTEM WILL KEEP TOXINS FROM LODGING IN YOUR BODY... KEEP IT CLEAN AND MOVING AND THE TOXINS DON'T HAVE

A CHANCE TO SINK IN, TAKE HOLD, DESTROY
YOUR BODY AND CAUSE DISEASE.'
– Harvey Diamond

As Harvey mentioned in his email to me, the 'One Disease – One Solution' hypothesis is a hard one for most to grasp, mainly because we have been almost programmed to treat the symptoms of illness and ignore the cause. If I have one main goal for this book, it's to hammer home just how blind most of us have become to the obvious. We have been blinded by science and blinded by people in white coats, people whom we immediately trust to know what's right. But as I have mentioned in the introduction, and as I will be expanding on a little later in the book, history has taught us that the people in white coats, holding clipboards and armed with the latest scientific data don't always get it right.

Keep It Simple

I honestly believe the whole business of health/disease has been so incredibly overcomplicated and that the *vast majority* of ailments can be helped greatly by simply removing the rubbish coming in and replacing any nutritional deficiencies. Even as I say it, it seems so obvious it's a joke, and I cannot believe I suffered for years at the hands of disease without realizing it sooner. But the reason I didn't then realize what I now feel is so stupidly obvious is the same reason most people don't realize this. I had been conditioned since birth not to question the experts, especially when it comes to treating diseases. I had been taught to look at ways to treat the symptoms and not even consider at what could possibly be causing them.

If you're still finding the concept of 'One Disease – One Solution' hard to get your head around, I'd like to add a little illustration to the hypothesis. Come with me as we enter...

THE
GOLDFISH
BOWL

4

I use this example visually at my retreats, I used it briefly in my *7lbs in 7days Juice Master Diet* book, and it's a full animation in the film *Super Juice Me!* The reason for using it again here is because it is the easiest way to illustrate why you need to treat the body as a whole rather than trying to treat each apparently separate disease individually. I have used visuals here to help simplify even further what I am saying. I have done this not to dumb down or treat you like some sort of idiot, but because the brain tends to retain visual information better. Often we read something and forget it almost the second we finish the book. I make no apologies for the repetition in this book. The full understanding of my 'One Disease – One Solution' theory is of paramount importance if you are to jump onto the *Super Juice Me!* plan or try to convince a friend or family member to. Actually, you well may find yourself with a plastic goldfish and a bowl full of water trying to explain it to those you know in order to explain why you are dong this. Trust me, people's first reaction, even if you are overweight and ill and even if they are your loved ones, is one of, 'Why are you doing that? It sounds dangerous'. So, in order to convince them you haven't lost the plot, you may have your hands on a goldfish before you can say *Super Juice*

Me! Alternatively, you may, of course, just sit them down and show them the film. This usually does the trick.

However, even if you've seen the film yourself, as 'repetition is the mother of skill', it's worth revisiting 'The Goldfish Bowl' concept here.

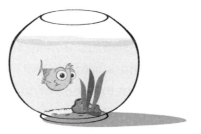

Here is a goldfish in a bowl of clean water with various plants.

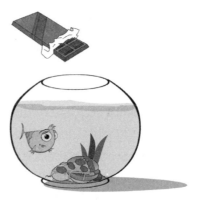

Now pour in a bag of white refined sugar; a load of refined fat, some chemical dyes, chemical flavourings, cigarettes, beer, white bread, caffeine, ice-cream, a few cakes, some donuts and other 'food'.

As the pollution enters the environment where the fish lives, the fish inevitably ingests a great deal of it. As the toxicity enters the fish's bloodstream its natural filtration system kicks in. Remember, survival comes first, health second. After a short period of time the toxicity begins to take its toll and the fish starts to get symptoms of dis-ease. A cough may begin, a few spots on its scales, it may get the mother of all headaches, perhaps it starts to bloat up, and maybe it can no longer move its fins as arthritis sets in. As this continues, diabetes may manifest itself and perhaps some gout. You get the picture.

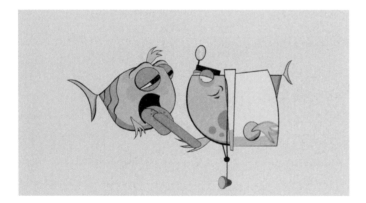

If the fish went to see a pharmacist or doctor, what would be the usual approach to helping the fish and the many apparently 'different' ailments it has? Drugs! Perhaps a little drug-based cough medicine to ease the cough. Maybe some insulin tablets to help cope with the Type 2 diabetes, a little cortisone injection to get the fins moving again, a few aspirins for the headaches, maybe even a quick operation to fit a gastric lap-band to prevent the fish from getting any bigger, or some new wonder-drug weight-loss pills, and let's not forget some steroid based cream to help with the itchy and flaky spots forming all over the surface of the fish. All of this then gets added to the bowl.

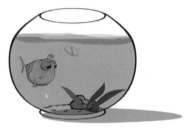

'THE DRUGS DON'T WORK, THEY JUST MAKE IT WORSE'
–THE VERVE

It is worth knowing that *all* drugs are also poisons and are *all* toxic to some degree to the body. This of course only *adds* to the overall pollution. The fish 'feels' better with the drugs, as now it can breath and move, it doesn't have a headache and its skin doesn't itch. It can also continue to eat the crap in the bowl, to which it has now become addicted, because it is taking pills to keep it 'slim' and 'well'. Clearly, the *cause* of every single ailment and disease the fish is suffering from hasn't been addressed one iota. Not only has it not been addressed, but the many toxic drugs entering the bowl are *adding* to the overall pollution, making it harder for the fish's natural filtration system to do its job effectively.

It doesn't take someone with a PhD or Bachelor's degree in medical science to figure out why the fish is sick, nor why it's continuing to experience more and more 'different' illnesses and symptoms. It also doesn't require Sherlock Holmes to figure out what is needed to help the fish. I have given this talk in schools to children as young as 10. When I ask the children what they would do, the only answer that comes screaming back very loudly is:

CLEAN THE WATER!

Yes, the only logical and common sense approach is to stop the pollution and clean the water. But, as I mentioned at the start of this book, common sense isn't that common, and there is simply far too much money in BIG PHARMA to begin to contemplate something as simple as stopping the pollution and cleaning the water as a solution to any common ailment or lifestyle disease.

I have already mentioned that short-term medical intervention is often absolutely necessary, but it should be just that – short-term. It should be a *short-term* solution until we get to the *cause* of the problem. Long-term medical drug use should only be given in the most extreme *minority* of cases and only when absolutely necessary, when all other natural methods have been exhausted or it is too late for natural treatments. Some people clearly do need medication for life. However, what we shouldn't have is a situation where the *first* point of call at the *first* sign of a few symptoms is a prescription for medical drugs. However, the sad truth remains that as long as there are billions of dollars at stake, drug therapy will always remain the first point of call for treatment, even if it doesn't make common sense and even if there are sometimes horrific – and in some cases deadly – side effects. The sheer volume of medical drugs being prescribed daily has now reached epidemic proportions. We need to understand that drugs of any kind, legal or illegal, are extremely big business and nothing comes as big in the legal drug world as...

BIG PHARMA

IT OFTEN DOESN'T MAKE SENSE BUT IT MAKES A LOT OF $$$$

5

I must make myself clear. I am not talking about *emergency* medical intervention, which will always be 100 per cent necessary. I am talking about this 'pill for every ill and an ill for every pill' society that has been created by the pharmaceutical industry on the back of people's fear. Fear, let's not forget, that is created by BIG PHARMA in the first place. I am talking about this mad world where people are popping pills for decades – not weeks, decades! Toxic medical drugs going into the bloodstream *every single day*, year upon year, with no end in sight. Things have now become so bad with BIG PHARMA that people are being encouraged to take a cocktail of different drugs *just in case* they get ill one day. You read that correctly: they are putting the fear of God into people by telling them that, unless they take this or that drug *while they are healthy*, they will, in the future, suffer this or that disease. And such is the power of persuasion by BIG PHARMA and their ability to use fear as a driving force for sales that people are doing this without even a single question!

Ask someone to fill in their family history and then tell them, 'There's a 10 per cent chance that you'll get heart disease, so take this pill for life,' and, boom, they'll take it! How do you even accurately calculate a 10 per cent risk of any disease? If there were a 10 per cent chance it would rain tomorrow, I'd leave the umbrella at home. Yet at the time of writing this book, BIG PHARMA have somehow convinced the UK government that everyone with as a little as a 10 ten per cent risk of coronary heart disease (CHD) should be on statins (cholesterol-lowering drugs) for life! I honestly wish I were making this up, but there's a lot – and I mean a *lot* – of money in pharmaceutical drugs, especially when the NHS (the UK's National Health Service) give them the nod.

F.E.A.R
FALSE EVIDENCE THAT APPEARS REAL

There is a massive difference between short-term medical emergencies and this long-term BIG PHARMA racket. And that is precisely what it is – a bloody racket. It's a racket built out of people's fears and insecurities. It's the fear BIG PHARMA create from the scientific 'evidence' *they* have usually, in some way or another, funded, and from the white coats they wear. They have instilled this fear by telling us we'll die prematurely or suffer a life of ill health unless we start taking this or that drug. They are now even putting this fear into people who are currently in tip-top condition.

How have we reached the stage where it is deemed to be not only reasonable but good practice for otherwise healthy people to have the fear of premature death put into them in order for a company to sell drugs and boost their share price for their investors? This is never how it's put, of course.

After all, it's all part of 'the war on disease', a war in which you can seemingly justify almost anything, a war which in reality many in BIG PHARMA don't actually want to win. The real money after all lies in 'the lifetime value of a customer'. *Repeat* prescriptions for life are what the shareholders are after. Let's not forget these drug companies are PLCs (Public Limited Companies) and ironically, they have *by law* to do what they can to increase profits for their shareholders. One sure-fire way of doing such a thing is to make sure that the end user is on that drug for life. Go one stage further and start giving drugs to healthy people 'just in case' and you have just widened the drug market to millions more whilst keeping the shareholders very, very happy.

I often wonder what actually would happen if a drug company did manage to produce a pill that cured every disease on earth in a day for virtually no money. Would they be breaking the law because they were longer increasing profits for the shareholders after the first year?

BIG PHARMA love lifestyle diseases because they can use the pills to treat the symptoms daily, giving the impression they are doing something worthwhile whilst never getting to the cause. All of which leads nicely to what seems to be what appears to be their 'pills for life' campaign.

Disease causes fear, and many in BIG PHARMA want to prey on that fear and even create fear that isn't there. The new fear they are creating, quite successfully I may add, is that, even as a healthy individual, you may be at risk unless you take their new wonder drug. They don't claim you won't get this or that health issue by taking this new pill, but they can show you 'proof' that they can lower the risk for you. This means they are always covered and essentially can never be proved wrong or held accountable. If you get the disease even when taking their wonder drug, well it happens. If you don't get the disease it's now because of the drug – genius!

I feel long-term medical drug use is rarely needed for the vast majority of people with lifestyle diseases, and it is, I feel, never required for those who are otherwise healthy. Why would anyone in their right mind give a healthy person medical drugs, which all have adverse side-effects to some degree, every day for life 'just in case' something happens? Perhaps I should cut my head off as a cure for any future headaches.

There are now things called 'polypills', a cocktail of several medical drugs all thrown into one. These are being hailed as the new all-singing and all-dancing treatment and prevention aid. They usually consist usually of five drugs in one: a statin, an aspirin and three blood-pressure medicines. The polypill was developed because the average older person takes an average of five pills a day for various conditions. The pharmaceutical companies argue that the more medicines a person takes, the more likely they are to forget to take one, so they've come up with the polypill. They didn't stop to ask why on earth the average older person is taking five medical pills a day. How has that now become the norm? How is it the norm, when all that's needed is often a few simple dietary changes? Scurvy killed thousands of people years ago, yet all that was required to cure this disease was a simple lime. If scurvy was a newly discovered disease, I guarantee BIG PHARMA would be all over it like a rash. They'd quickly see that it's a simple case of a vitamin C deficiency, but they'd produce papers and studies making it far more complicated than it really is, and they'd recommend to the NHS that everyone should be taking their patented 'scurvy prevention pill' daily for life to remove any risk of getting it.

The crazy thing is, if you did have scurvy and I told you to skip their drug because I could cure scurvy with a simple lemon or a lime, I would be charged with 'practising medicine without a licence'. And that is what is happening today. For example, it has been shown that apples and their juice can help lower cholesterol, but when was the last time you heard of any doctor saying, 'Skip the statins, have an apple'? There are much, much better ways of lowering cholesterol than a cholesterol-lowering drug. I have seen people drop 2 points in just 7 days on a juice-only diet, but all you hear is how 'juicing is dangerous'. The last thing they want is for the vast majority of us to wake up and realize that the majority of lifestyle disease doesn't require a cocktail of medical drugs but a lifestyle change – one that's in our own hands with no adverse side-effects.

BEWARE! ALTERNATIVE 'MEDICINE' IS SNAKE OIL

And that's the other area where BIG PHARMA prey on our fears and insecurities to keep the drug merry-go-round churning away. They make certain an even greater fear is created if you dare even think about seeking anything other than medical drugs to treat your ills. I have been called a 'snake-oil salesman' more times than I care to mention. It appears that those who suggest a non-medical approach for disease are pretty much all tarnished with the same snake-oily brush. No doubt if scurvy was the new disease on the block and BIG PHARMA had a pill to 'cure' and 'prevent' it (a pill which would clearly contain vitamin C but which would also include a whole bunch of other stuff so they could call it a drug and patent it), and if I said, 'A lime does the same thing, so stop taking the drug,' I'd be in prison! I would also be deemed a 'snake-pill salesman' if I were selling lemons and limes. BIG PHARMA would make sure that *you* believed their drug contained vital other elements that a simple lime doesn't. They would scare the life out of you if you even contemplated taking the non-patented no-prescription-needed lime instead of their wonder drug. They would produce scientific evidence about their pill and find examples of where someone who had simply relied on a lime had perished. They wouldn't have perished because of the lime or because of scurvy; the lime would have prevented that. But any link to this person's dying prematurely because they choose to lime-it rather than drug-it would be used to scare you into never seeking 'alternative' ways to treat any ills. The message is clear: BIG PHARMA knows best so stick with us and you'll be fine and dandy.

On one thing I do agree with BIG PHARMA and that is that there are many, many 'snake-oil salespeople' out there. More needs to be done to crack down on them. I was a victim of many myself, when seeking other ways to treat my psoriasis, asthma, eczema and hay fever. The amount I spent on the internet ordering 'amazing creams' for my psoriasis at stupid money added up to thousands. None of the creams worked and the only thing they cleared up was my bank account, not my skin. I wholeheartedly agree that these people need closing down; they prey on people's insecurities and desperation.

However, there's a very big difference between someone passing off bog-standard moisturizing cream as a 'cure' for psoriasis and what I am talking about here. The 'One Disease – One Solution' approach is about removing the toxic rubbish coming into the body and replacing any nutrient deficiencies with the natural nutrient-packed juices which flow within every fruit and vegetable, juices which, by design, were meant to act as both food *and* medicine, juices that are effectively feeders *and* healers. You cannot possibly put natural juice therapy or plant food therapy in the same bracket as the pretend pills and potions that promise miracle cures, which are littering the internet as we speak.

The problem is that BIG PHARMA do put the two in the same bracket as the last thing they want or need is the sudden realization that the solution for your ills may be just as close as your kitchen. But they know that even if you begin to believe such a thing, which intuitively makes sense – after all it is hard to argue against the simplicity of GOLDFISH BOWL analogy – their task is to create enough fear so that you won't ever trust that intuition. It's all about trusting only those in the white coats, who do the 'scientific studies' that confirm how wonderful their drugs are. To go elsewhere is foolhardy at best and it's 'at your own risk, but you have been warned'.

I wouldn't mind if what BIG PHARMA were offering did the trick. I'd be right behind them every step of the way. I wouldn't mind if it was the solution for lifestyle diseases, but it clearly isn't working in the way or to the extent they claim.

You could even argue that much of BIG PHARMA resemble the very 'snake-oil salespeople' they claim you need to steer well clear of. On the day I am writing this very page, another 'wonder' drug has hit the national headlines. This time the headline reads,

'Drug that could curb urge to shop'

I thought I had seen it all until I read this. BIG PHARMA want you to believe there is a pill for literally everything, even shopping too much! Not only do they have the 'a pill for every ill' mantra, as I have already touched on, but also 'an *ill* for every pill'. This is where they effectively change the illness a particular drug is best suited for. One example is Zyban. Zyban was originally an anti depressant drug, but because some people stopped smoking whilst using it, it then got rebadged as an anti-smoking drug. The same, it appears, is happening with this new wonder drug that can apparently 'curb your urge to shop'. The drug they are testing on the human guinea pigs that like to shop a little too much or who have 'compulsive buying disorder', as it's called, is an epilepsy drug. This way they don't need to go through the huge time and expense of getting a new drug approved for this shopping 'disorder', because it's not a new drug, it's just a new use for that drug!

Your brain is your 'head office', if you will; everything passes through and it controls everything. I have no idea what possible side effects you could get by giving a person who over-shops an epilepsy drug. And neither do they! If their 'scientific research' is 'successful' – by showing that the people who took part in the trial shop less, I guess – then millions of people all over the world could soon be popping these pills in a bid to 'curb the urge to shop'.

The biggest issue I have is not just that these drugs change the make-up of a person's brain chemistry in ways they don't always know, given the billions of different connections made every second in the brain, but that in their bid to produce more and more drugs, BIG PHARMA keep coming up with more and more random 'disorders'. It appears that we soon won't have to take personal responsibility for anything, as we'll all have a medical psychological 'disorder' of some kind. When did excess shopping become a medical disorder? More importantly, when did we reach a situation where it's accepted as perfectly normal to pop a medical pill for just about everything? And when did it become OK for the medical profession to make up names for supposed new conditions and then tell people that the best way to curb their 'disorder' is to change their brain chemistry with this new 'breakthrough' medical drug? The expression 'blinded by science' appears to be alive and well when it comes to finding new uses for existing drugs and inventing disorders that require a pill.

TRUST IN CONVENTIONAL MEDICINE
...we've done the science to back it up!

The difference between 'alternative' and 'conventional' medicine, we are told, is just how strictly conventional medicine is governed. Supposedly only drugs that have been cleared as 'safe' with stringent scientific backing are approved by the Medicines and Healthcare Products Regulatory Agency

(MHRA) in the UK or by the Federal Drugs Administration (FDA) in the USA.

However, I have just done a little research and found 35 medical drugs which have been taken off the market since 1970 because they cause more problems than they solve. Some of those 'problems' aren't slight; they include death, which is about as severe a side effect as you can get! I am sure there are more than the 35 I've found and I'm not going to list them all here – that would be a book in itself – but it's worth pointing out a couple. Please remember these were all approved and all had 'good' scientific backing, proving their effectiveness.

Diethylstibestrol

Uses: Synthetic oestrogen to prevent miscarriage, premature labour, and other pregnancy complications
On the market: 31 years
Removed from the market: 1971 in the USA
Reasons it was removed from the market: Clear cell adenocarcinoma (cancer of the cervix and vagina), birth defects, and other developmental abnormalities in children born to women who took the drug while pregnant; increased risk of breast cancer, higher risk of death from breast cancer; risk of cancer in children of mothers taking the drug including raised .risk of breast cancer after age 40; increased risk of fertility and pregnancy complications, early menopause, testicular abnormalities; potential risks for third generation children (the grandchildren of women who took the drug) but they are unclear as

studies are just beginning.

Studies in the 1950s showed the drug was not effective at preventing miscarriages, premature labour, or other pregnancy complications.

★   ★   ★

Selacryn (Tienilic acid)

Use: Hypertension (blood pressure)
Manufacturer: SmithKline
On the market: 3 years
Removed from the market: 1982
Reasons it was removed from the market: Hepatitis: 36 deaths. At least 500 cases of severe liver and kidney damage.

Anphar Labs, who developed the drug in France and sold US marketing rights to SmithKline, reported to SmithKline in April 1979 (translated in May 1979 to English from French) that Selacryn was associated with liver damage. On December 13, 1984, SmithKline Beckman pleaded guilty in a US court to, '14 counts of failing to file reports with the drug agency of adverse reactions to Selacryn and 20 counts of falsely labeling the drug with a statement that there was no known cause-and-effect relationship between Selacryn and liver damage'.

★   ★   ★

Vioxx (Rofecoxib)

Use: Non-steroidal anti-inflammatory drug for pain relief.

Manufacturer: Merck

On the market: 5.3 years

Removed from the market: September 30, 2004

Reasons it was removed from the market: Increased risk of heart attack and stroke; linked to about 27,785 heart attacks or sudden cardiac deaths between May 20, 1999 and 2003.

Ads for Vioxx features Olympic gold medallists Dorothy Hamill and Bruce Jenner. Vioxx was prescribed to more than 20 million people.

There are loads more, but we don't have time here and you get the picture. Vioxx was perhaps the most famous recall of a drug in recent years, due to the sheer numbers of associated deaths. Note that these are the ones that were actually recalled; and don't forget some drugs are on the market for decades before they are pulled from the market. BIG PHARMA do the maths and have a 'law suit' contingency budget plan set aside for when – not if – one of their drugs is shown to cause horrific side effects and people start suing. They simply look at what they pay out overall compared to revenue the drug brings in. Providing the latter is the larger figure, they remain happy campers.

You see, despite the almost 30,000 deaths (actually that figure is now believed to be around 55,000, but no one will ever truly know the extent) linked to Vioxx, it only ever costs the BIG PHARMA company money, not time in the clink. If 30,000 people died on my juice retreat, I somehow feel I'd be looking at the world from behind bars. Even when it was proved that the drug company in question knew before the drug was launched in 1999 that it could cause possible strokes and heart attacks, not one person went to prison – not one!

We simply have no way of knowing what drugs that are on the market right now are truly safe. It could take years before we know the truth. BIG PHARMA is BIG BUSINESS. If they can sweep the horrific side-effects of a drug like Vioxx under the table before it's launched, what's to prevent them doing it again? Please also remember these are single drugs we are talking about here. What happens when you become a walking drug experiment with a cocktail of things swimming in your bloodstream every day?

THE BIG DRUG EXPERIMENT

Take Andy Morris for example, the Welsh guy who was in the film *Super Juice Me!* Andy turned up for the *Super Juice Me! Big Juice Experiment* with two suitcases. One had clothes, as you'd expect, but the other was entirely full of drugs. This is no exaggeration. If you've seen the film you will know this. If you haven't yet seen the film it will blow your mind. This man had a list of diseases as long as your arm and list of drugs to match. He was taking 62 tablets a day – every day! That's 62 MEDICAL DRUG PILLS EVERY SINGLE DAY. Or, to put it another way, OVER 1,700 TABLETS A MONTH. This would be all fine and dandy if he was in fine fettle and was the picture of health, but the drugs were simply keeping him in a zombie-type state and creating a multitude of side effects and addiction. One of the funniest moments of the film is when Andy starts to read the side effects of the drugs he's on. It's a priceless moment in the film and sums up for me the madness of it all. He estimates that 80 per cent of the medical drugs he was taking were to try to counter the side effects of the other 20 per cent he apparently had to have. I think that's worth repeating and shouting about. It's too easy to pass such things without much thought:

80 PER CENT OF THE DRUGS HE WAS TAKING WERE TO TRY AND COUNTER THE SIDE EFFECTS CAUSED BY THE OTHER 20 PER CENT OF DRUGS HE ACTUALLY NEEDED

This is about as brilliant as a business model gets. You prescribe someone a few drugs with the full knowledge you'll get an 80 per cent 'up-sell' soon after because of the side-effects you know the drugs you have given them will cause. Genius!

Can you take someone like Andy off of those drugs overnight? NO! Not once he's in to that extent. He's now so heavily addicted and dependent on them that the withdrawal alone would be far too dangerous. But what you can do for him is at least to start to 'clean the water', and then gradually, as the body starts to heal itself, it is highly probable that some of those drugs can be reduced or even eliminated altogether. One thing is for sure: he can't possibly get well by continuing to take a suitcase full of toxic pills

for life. This isn't getting to the cause of any of his genuine
health issues; it's putting sticky plasters over them at best.
The pills do nothing whatsoever to clean the environment
where his cells 'bathe', if you will, and they ultimately add to
the pollution. Clean the pollution and you have the chance
at least of one happy and healthier fish!

> Dear Jason
>   … I was on 19 tablets a day for pain, high blood
> pressure, high cholesterol and depression, I had also been
> diagnosed as having emphysema. I was told if I continued
> as I was I had a high chance of a heart attack. Then you
> came back into my life… I am presently on day 38 of 60
> of a juice fast… I am now TOTALLY off all pills. YES that's
> 570 pills a month I am no longer taking. I took myself off
> them and at first my doctor was not impressed but being
> open minded continues to take my blood pressure and
> check my blood etc and readily admits seldom has she
> seen such a turnaround in a person's health…

The above is just a snippet from a long letter I received. This
part is relevant here. I have received many of the same ilk,
and once again it illustrates beautifully how the body wants
to heal, given the chance to do so. It also shows once again
how medical drugs are dished out so readily. This man was
taking 570 tablets a month. How is that even right? He's far
from alone. There are thousands, if not millions, all over the
world taking a cocktail of pills every day, and the craziest
thing about it all is that it's seen as normal. It is so far from
normal it's a joke. In the film, I mention that my one goal

above all is to stop people rattling. You pick up the average person, especially in the US, and shake them and they'll rattle! The quantity of medical drugs being dished out is, in my opinion, way out of control.

Giving a cocktail, or, in Andy's case, an entire suitcase of medical drugs to people who have what are deemed to be many different diseases, is one thing. But I find it absurd and almost criminal to be giving liver-toxic, side-effect-heavy, medical drugs daily to otherwise healthy people, which is what is happening right now. Giving drugs to Andy now that he's in this position – largely caused by the drugs themselves – needs addressing in the way I have described and in the way we tackled it in the film. Ironically, some of those drugs, given Andy's diet and lack of exercise may well be keeping him alive. Until the 'water' is clean he needs at least some of them. However, to dish out medical drugs to otherwise healthy people is utterly insane.

And before anyone from the medical profession who is reading this feels I'm giving dangerous advice, I am not talking about not giving someone malaria tablets when travelling to a country where that disease is endemic. Clearly I'm not against that, as it's an intelligent use of medical drugs. Clearly you give those to a healthy person for protection whilst they are away, but it's very, very short-term and there's a good reason for it. You wouldn't give the person malaria tablets for life once they return to the UK 'just in case' they bumped into someone who had it, would you? You simply cannot argue that giving a healthy person a drug, like a statin, every day for life, when that person is 100 per cent healthy, is an intelligent thing to do. Well, I say you cannot argue, but using 'scientific' research they do argue this. It's that very same 'scientific' research which helps the fear factor and makes most people extremely reluctant to go down any other route than medical drugs. We are conditioned to believe a medical pill can do so much to treat disease, but that fruits and vegetables cannot.

The scary thing is Andy represents just one of millions like him. It's one of the reasons BIG PHARMA have the slickest offices and biggest bonus structures in the world. In the US BIG PHARMA are so prolific that it is legal for them to advertise their prescription drugs on TV, something still not allowed in Europe. Every time I'm in the US I am amazed at the medical pill knowledge of the average person in the street. They know the longest names for just about every famous medical drug and exactly what it is 'good' for. The adverts always list a load of symptoms and ask the viewer such questions as 'Do you suffer with any of the following…? If so, help is at hand with our all-singing and all-dancing drug.' The list of symptoms they give out are like fortune tellers' Tarot cards (sorry if you're into them!) in that they will always relate to you in some way. For example, put an advert on TV in the daytime and say 'Do you suffer with back pain?', and, as the average day time viewer is around 50-70 years old, the chances are they will answer the question with a big YES. Why? because the drug companies know that most people of that age have back issues of some kind. It's worth knowing that 98 per cent of people have a back problem at some stage before they pass. This is all these companies want you to do, say a sub-conscious 'yes' – as your brain will – then accept that what they are offering will help this problem for *you*.

Put out another ad asking people if they ever suffer from bloating, indigestion, nausea, skin irritation and so on and, boom, you've got almost everyone. The advert then shows you images of a family dancing in a field, holding hands and being happy, all because of the drug. The drug has saved a family member from this or that and now they are free to be themselves with their loved ones again. All of this while you conveniently ignore the long list of possible side-effects that are voiced by the fastest talker in the world!

This is all designed of course to get the person watching to go to their doctor and demand that particular make of drug. Doctors, especially in the US, are BIG PHARMA's biggest 'customers'. BIG PHARMA will do almost anything to convince that doctor to push their particular drug over its competitors. Fancy a five-star all-expenses-paid trip to Hawaii for a 'conference', Mr Doctor? No worries, we have it covered!

BIG FAT PROFITS

Cholesterol-lowering drugs are BIG PHARMA's golden egg at the moment. Weight-loss tablets are on a level playing field with the statins and are also big business. Unfortunately, whereas you once could only get a weight loss pill if it was prescribed by your doctor, now anyone can freely buy one over the counter at any pharmacy. They claim that not everyone can buy one and that you need to have a particular BMI (Body Mass Index), but anyone can jump online, make up their BMI number and get these weight loss tablets sent to their door. As with any medical drug, there are side effects.

Now I have read many lists of drugs' side effect lists in my life; many of these are somewhat ironic, such as 'may cause suicidal thoughts' on anti-depressant pills. Sadly the irony with that one seems to have flown over many heads.

I have yet to read one more hilarious than one side effect of a certain weight-loss pill. Most weight-loss pills 'work' by trapping the fat you eat and removing it from the body without its being digested. Most concentrate on this as they are still under the incredibly false apprehension that it's FAT that makes you fat. This all comes from a study by a guy called Ancel Keys, who linked dietary fat to making people fat and ill. I've somewhat simplified that, clearly, but essentially it sums it up. This study led to the massive anti-fat propaganda which has been going on for years and is only just starting to subside. Only now are people starting to realize that refined sugar and refined fat are the issue. However, most still believe in the 'fat makes you fat' hypothesis and this is what BIG PHARMA play on when producing their anti-fat pills. It's why they concentrate on trapping the fat you eat and disposing of it before it's digested. However, there are a few major flaws to this, such as the failure to absorb any fat-soluble vitamins and, of course, the fact that ultimately these pills are about as effective as Tony Blair as a peace keeper. However, the biggest problem is the main side effect. I read and re-read it, thinking I must be seeing things. It stated, 'Watch out for unannounced anal leakage'; that's...

UNANNOUNCED!

That is one area where I'd like as much warning as possible! How the blazes have we reached this stage in human development and health care, where we are popping medical pills that make us crap ourselves – unannounced let's not forget – rather than eating some fruit? You even can 'add to basket' a pair of pants to go with the drugs to take care of your 'anal leakage' (no I am not kidding). How do we think this is remotely normal and, moreover, how the hell do so many medics prescribe this stuff whilst at the same time saying that fresh juice diets are dangerous? Please excuse the rather crass abbreviation here but…WTF!

What I also love about these weight-loss pills is that they come with a disclaimer stating that they are 'only effective in conjunction with diet and exercise'. I find this particularly odd, given that many medics will stress that these pills are useful for many people when other methods have failed them. What, like diet and exercise? If they're designed for people who cannot achieve their goal through diet and exercise and yet claim they are only effective with diet and exercise, how can they possibly work?

WHEN IN DOUBT
CUT IT OUT!

However, no need to worry, because, if all else fails, simply cut it out. Bariatric surgery is now huge business. Between April 2006 and March 2012 there were 18,577 gastric-bypass and 7,650 gastric-band operations, costing the NHS over £85 million! In 2006-7 there were 858 gastric bypass operations carried out in the UK by the NHS, but just six years later that figure went up to 5,407 – a six-fold increase in just six years. And this figure doesn't include anyone who went private, which runs into many thousands more.

All of this expenditure would be justified if this approach was working, but it isn't. I have personally met people who have undergone such operations and who remain overweight and extremely ill, often much sicker than before the operation. Many people have reported that it's easy to cheat the system by simply blending things like chocolate with Coke and drinking it! These are not just my own observations either. More and more people are questioning the effectiveness of this type of expensive and *extremely* drastic surgery. One study by Dutch doctors found that the success rate for gastric banding might be so low that it calls into question whether the operation is worth doing. Five years after surgery a third failed to lose significant weight; after 10 years, two-thirds were around their original size. As a result of complications, a third of patients needed the operation re-done after five years, while half needed this at 10 years.

'YOU MUST REALISE THIS IS NOT THE FINAL ANSWER MOST OF THE TIME.'
– LEAD RESEARCHER DR EDO AARTS

These aren't the only issues. Research is now pointing to long-term health problems, including bone thinning, fractures, anaemia, kidney stones, and psychological problems, even suicide.

As with any major surgery, the risks of having a gastric

bypass can prove fatal. Over just a three-year period, 29 people died as a direct result of these operations. Thirty-year-old Kerry Greaves was one of them. Kerry died after an operation to fit a gastric band went wrong. Kerry suffered complications soon after a gastric bypass operation and died a month later. Doctors tried operating 14 times to try to save her. Her stomach was leaking bile and she died from organ failure. Kerry was 18st (252lbs) and wanted surgical help to slim because she feared her daughter would be bullied 'for having a fat mum'. Don't get me wrong, 18st isn't slim or healthy, but I have dealt with people a lot heavier and there is no way, in my opinion, she should have ever been allowed surgery in the first place. Who in the medical profession thought this operation was her very last resort?

Kerry's mother, Anne, warned, 'My advice to anybody thinking of having this operation would be: "Have more pride in yourself and don't do it."'

I could put each and every tragic story into this chapter to add a little human emotion to the numbers, but we don't have time. Kerry was just 30 years young when somebody somewhere with good medical credentials signed a piece of paper which ultimately led to her passing. If there were 29 deaths at my 'Juice Camp' in three years, I'd be shut down before you could even say 'Super Juice Me!' Actually that's not true. If I had just one person die whilst at the juice camp as a direct result of the 'alternative' treatment they were on, I would be shut down. Add a prison sentence to that, shock headlines in all newspapers and the lead story on Sky News, then we get close to what would actually happen. Yet when deaths occur in the medical world as a direct result of the treatment they advise, it's all considered 'collateral damage' in the war on disease and obesity.

BOY, AGED TWO, HAS FAT OP

When I saw the above headline, I honestly thought it must be an April Fools joke, but it was September and it was far from a joke. A Saudi Arabian two-year-old boy who weighed 5st (70lbs) had 70 per cent of his stomach removed to help him lose weight. Let's understand this correctly, doctors put a *two-year-old* child under anaesthetic and removed 70 per cent of his stomach because 'two attempts at dieting had failed' and it was 'a last resort'. Now call me 'Mr Are You Flipping Kidding Me', but am I missing something here? How on earth does a two-year-old 'fail' at a diet? Did his mates call up at the weekend and suggest a few drinks and a dinner party he just couldn't resist? Did he get dressed at 2am to nip to the local garage because he just had to have some chocolate and crisps? HE'S TWO! Not 22. Where can he go without the help of others? Who is feeding the kid? Maybe – and just a wild idea here – instead of ripping out 70 per cent of this two year old's stomach so he'll eat less, a better plan would be to simply restrict what he ate by **NOT GIVING HIM THE EXCESS FOOD!** Radical, I know.

Seriously though, how was this operation even legal? Diets cannot fail on a two year old; it's impossible. Are they suggesting that they actually restricted this boys intake by putting him on a diet, but he still piled on the pounds? If that was the justification for taking such drastic and dangerous measures, then it's still flawed. The operation is all about restricting the amount the boy eats, which is the same as a diet. If apparently restricting his intake via dieting didn't work, then how will the surgery?

As it turns out the boy lost 18lbs within two months after the operation, proving that restriction of food intake works a treat. Funny that! It transpires that dieting would have indeed worked and he wasn't 'big boned' and he didn't have a 'slow metabolism'! Rip out 70 per cent of a two-year-old's stomach and all is well on the medical front, but suggest that someone who is overweight and ill should live on freshly extracted fruit and vegetable juices for 28 days and you're attacked as doing something dangerous. Given the choice between the two options I know which one I'd pick every single time – show me the juice!

And why didn't they simply give this kid some of the 'amazing' weight-loss pills which have been 'proven' to be so effective? Surely a few pills would have been a better option than the removal of a considerable chunk of the child's stomach? Why didn't they use the fat pills? BECAUSE THEY DON'T WORK. It's all part of the 'Big Pharma Illusion Show', where misdirection combines with fear to have us all blindly taking pills and getting bits of us cut out without ever really questioning it. It's where many are hoodwinked into believing the medical way is the only way and all other approaches are dangerous and should be treated with great caution. The biggest irony of course is that it's often the medical approach we need to treat with great caution.

THE USA SPENDS MORE ON MEDICAL HEALTH CARE THAN ANY OTHER COUNTRY IN THE WORLD,

YET REMAINS ONE OF THE SICKEST

The USA alone spends $2.8 trillion on health care each year, fat pills included. To put this into perspective, if the health-care system were to break off from the United States and become its own economy it would be the fifth largest in the world. It would be bigger than the UK and France. You would think that, if were its own economy and we made it into its own private country you'd have the healthiest country on earth. Yet despite spending $2.8 trillion, at the end of each year the USA becomes a sicker nation than it was the year before. Not only are the vast majority of these drugs not making us better, but they are often adding to the death toll.

Many years ago Professor Bruce Pomerance of the University of Toronto concluded that properly prescribed and correctly prescribed and correctly taken pharmaceutical drugs were the fourth leading cause of death in the US. Let me repeat that again, because it's easy to let certain things pass over you when reading:

PROPERLY PRESCRIBED AND CORRECTLY PRESCRIBED AND CORRECTLY TAKEN PHARMACEUTICAL DRUGS WERE THE FOURTH LEADING CAUSE OF DEATH IN THE US

However, that was years ago and things have changed, but not for the better. In the health film *Food Matters* it was stated that properly prescribed and correctly taken medical drugs are now the *third* leading cause of death in the US.

ADVERSE DRUG REACTIONS AND MEDICAL ERRORS NOW ACCOUNT FOR OVER ONE HUNDRED THOUSAND DEATHS IN THE USA ALONE ... *ANNUALLY!*

I want to be clear here. This figure is not for overdoses or misuse of those drugs; this figure is based on 'drugs used as directed'. Once again all of this gets put down to 'collateral damage' in the 'war on disease'. It's not only adverse drug reactions causing collateral damage either. Deaths caused by errors in hospital are somewhat mind-blowing too. In 1999 the Institute of Medicine (IOM) published a seminal report titled *To Err is Human*, which estimated that at least 44,000 patients — and probably as many as 98,000 — die in hospitals each year as results of medical errors.

DEATHS FROM MEDICAL ERRORS ARE EQUIVALENT TO 10 JUMBO JETS CRASHING EACH WEEK

A follow-up study published in 2013 argued that the IOM numbers were a vast underestimate and that medical errors contribute to the deaths of between 210,000 and 440,000 patients. At the lower bound that's the equivalent of nearly 10 jumbo jets crashing every week.

When I was 15 years old, my mother went to hospital with a cyst the size of an orange on one of her ovaries. She was told they would need to remove the ovary. This was bad enough news in itself, but far worse was to come when, after the operation, they discovered they had accidentally removed the wrong ovary! I had to leave school at 15 and find a job pronto to support my mother and me, as she was now in bed.

Fast forward a couple of decades. She went back to the doctors on more than one occasion, complaining of breathing difficulties and tightness in the chest. After several appointments and check-ups, they came to the conclusion she had COPD – Chronic Obstructive Pulmonary Disease – and prescribed an asthma pump. It turned out she had lung cancer, which was left untreated because of the misdiagnosis for four long years – enough time to for it to spread like wild-fire. It was an 'alternative' practitioner, funnily enough, who noticed her finger nails were bent over and said, 'You need to get that checked out. I think you've got either TB or cancer.' (I bet you're looking at your nails now, right?) Off my mother popped to the doctor to get it properly checked out and, sure enough, it was cancer.

I say cancer, but it wasn't just cancer. It was stage four 'you've got six months left to live' type of cancer. I'd say that's the worst kind. It was the 'sorry there's nothing we can do' type of cancer. It was the kind of cancer which broccoli juice doesn't really stand a chance against!

The reason for mentioning such facts is not to put you off going into hospital, taking medical drugs or having operations. All of these things are vital at times. The *intention* of every medic who saw my mother, diagnosed her or operated and took out the wrong ovary, was never one of malice. I honestly don't think any medic is in the business to harm or deliberately misdiagnose. But I believe quite a few in BIG PHARMA, especially those at the top, couldn't give a flying toss about anything other than profits for themselves and their shareholders and think, 'Let's take the collateral damage on the chin'. Conversely I think 99.99 per cent of doctors genuinely have the patient's best interest at heart. They may, in my opinion, go about it the wrong way on many occasions, but their intentions are good. Yes, clearly if the doctor in question had realized that my mother had lung cancer and not COPD way back when, I honestly believe my mother would be here today – early detection is after all the key. But his intention, which is everything, wasn't to do harm.

The reason I bring all of this to your attention is simply to point out that 'alternative medicine' doesn't have the luxury of the errors that conventional medicine does, or of any errors for that matter. If just one person ever died due to being on a juice diet, I'd not only be hammered but probably put on criminal charges, especially if I'd diagnosed the person.

Last year, I felt a little of what would occur should such a thing ever happen, when Bob Geldof's daughter Peaches died tragically at the tender age of just 25 years old. It was headline news that she had died because of her 'extreme' juice diet. The Daily Mail online led the way, and it was soon followed with the same global press headlines:

Speculation Rises Over Peaches Geldof's Extreme Juice Cleansing Habits In Relation To Her Death

This was just one of many headlines around the world. A well-known dietician in the UK who has attacked juice diets in the past, mine to be specific, was reported to have said

Peaches' diet was irresponsible and dangerous. As far as I am aware this dietician said this *before* Peaches had passed, and had never speculated that juicing had indeed been the cause of her death. Nonetheless, some newspapers and even TV shows leapt on her comments when trying to find a cause for her death. We need to remember that it was reported that there were no signs of drugs in Peaches' blood after death. This led to speculation elsewhere, about juicing to be precise. Here was just one of the headlines:

'... a spokesperson for the British Dietetic Association insists Geldof was "irresponsible to promote" the diet.'

The state registered dietician says, "Peaches joins a long line of celebs who are brain dead when it comes to nutrition. Surviving on fruit is a very dangerous diet. Peaches is at high risk of electrolyte abnormalities, which could lead to acute cardiac arrest.

"Rapid dieting like this not only makes you lose muscle strength but wastes away your internal organs. It is what kills anorexics. It is a stupid approach and it is irresponsible to promote this sort of disordered eating. It's worrying that somebody who has money and access to contacts would pick such a ridiculous way to diet."'

As far as I know, the dietician in question never once said that juicing caused Peaches' death or even implied it. All of her comments were made before Peaches passed. She did however say quite publicly state that Peaches was 'brain dead' when it came to nutrition, saying that surviving on fruit is a very dangerous diet. After the headlines started to appear it didn't take long before my Twitter and Facebook accounts were full of tweets and posts by trolls asking things like, 'How can you live with yourself?' and 'Look what your stupid diet has done, you've killed Peaches'. I wish I was joking, but no. This was the type of abuse I got after her tragic passing, all stimulated, I believe, by the ludicrous speculation she had died because she was on a juice diet. The speculation was fuelled to some degree by comments from qualified dieticians and doctors. As it turned out, Peaches tragically died because of a heroin overdose, not because of her consumption of fresh vegetable juice – shocker!

The point, however, is that nothing more that the speculation that one person may have died because of a juice diet (out of the *millions* of people who have done one), caused headlines around the world and personal attacks on me. Yet thousands upon thousands of people die from adverse medical drug reactions every year and it's just par for the course or 'collateral damage', as they put it.

Juicing can help millions of people, but heaven forbid that just one person ever has an adverse reaction to a juice diet. It would probably cause an immediate worldwide ban and certainly front-page news, as we have already found out!

THE ALTERNATIVE BLAME GAME

And that's another issue I have with the whole 'medical vs alternative' argument. If a person dies while undergoing medical treatment, it's claimed that it's the disease that killed them. If, on the other hand, a person refuses medical treatment and dies, it's now all of a sudden *because* they refused the medical treatment and chose an alternative. It now becomes the fault of the alternative treatment they are now taking, not the disease.

Take Jade Goody, for example. If you are reading this outside the UK and have never heard of her, Jade Goody became famous in the UK because of a show called *Big Brother*. Jade actually entered the Big Brother House twice, once in the 'normal' show and some years later in *Celebrity Big Brother*. Pretty soon after her appearance in *Celebrity Big Brother* she was diagnosed with quite aggressive cervical cancer. Through someone I knew who was good friends with her agent I contacted her agent and said I would happily do what I could to help, completely off the press radar (and I mentioned I would sign anything to that end too). Her agent said 'no thanks' and they had it all covered with 'real' medical help.

Now the point I wish to make is this: I am not saying for a nanosecond that if I had got involved and put her on some natural juice therapy she would have been saved. I am not saying that *at all*. You can never have a parallel universe, so there is never any way of knowing what would or would not have happened either way. My intention, just to be clear, would never have been to advise that she stopped any medical treatment but to do what I could do 'complement' it with freshly extracted vegetable juices. I am very much into complementary medicine. I honestly believe there is a place where *medical* and *alternative* therapies can complement each other and create the only type of medicine which makes sense, i.e. complementary. (I will explain more about this in the next chapter 'The Fire Brigade'.)

The point, though, is this: if her agent had said 'yes', and let's say Jade had decided to stop *all* medical intervention and go with only fresh juices as treatment, and say she had passed away on exactly the same date on which she did actually pass away, people's perceptions would have changed. No longer would it have been the cancer that had killed her but the fact she had agreed to see this quack with juice. See the difference?

Sadly Jade passed at a very young age and quite soon after diagnosis. She died despite the massive amount of medical help and treatment which became available to her and the many specialists who oversaw her treatment. It wasn't the drugs that killed her, it was, of course, the cancer. However, as mentioned, if she had died on exactly the same day while on juices in the absence of these experts and all the medical drug treatment, the reason for her death would have been heavily blamed on her having refused the medical treatment and chosen juices instead. I would essentially have been held to blame for being utterly irresponsible and I would have been blamed for her passing.

This is why BIG PHARMA & CO can never really fail. If they inadvertently kill someone as a direct result of an adverse side effect from a drug it's 'collateral damage', and in the 'war on disease' there's always going to be casualties so hey ho. And if someone dies of a disease like cancer while the medical profession throws everything they can at it, then it's the disease that kills them. It's nothing whatsoever to do with the type of treatment they tried. However, if you offer 'alternative' treatments and the disease still kills, YOU get the blame, not the disease. All of this helps to generate a fear of trying anything other than pharmaceutical medicine.

WE NEED TO CHANGE WHAT 'ALTERNATIVE' MEANS

I am unsure how we have reached the stage where fruits, vegetables, good air, exercise and a positive outlook are seen as an 'alternative' way to treat someone who is ill, while toxic medical drugs are deemed to be 'conventional', but we are where we are. When I was growing up, if someone was sick the first thing you thought of bringing them was a bowl of fruit. Not because you had been told that's what to do, but because *intuitively* you just kind of knew. There is a place for both kinds of treatment, medical and what's seen as 'alternative', but surely we need to switch it. If a person is unwell, then we should first seek to 'first do no harm' and give them water, rest and *good* nutrition. If that doesn't work, we should then seek an *alternative*, such as medical intervention.

Once again please do not misread or misquote what I am saying,

THERE WILL ALWAYS BE A NEED FOR PHARMACEUTICAL EMERGENCY HELP

There are many, even in BIG PHARMA, who do genuinely care and in times of a real disease emergency the medical approach is the *only* way one should go. I know this sounds a little contradictory from what I have said in this chapter, but pouring wheatgrass juice on a broken leg or eating some broccoli while you are actually having a heart attack is clearly never going to help! Equally, for ever popping pills for certain lifestyle diseases is never going to help in the long run either. There is a good solid need for both approaches, and each needs to be used at the right times for the right reasons and conditions. I believe drug-based therapy is completely unnecessary most of the time for many lifestyle diseases, but when there's an emergency the medical way is the *only* way. Or, to put it another way, and to once again use a visual analogy to help illustrate the point, there will always be times when we need to call in....

THE
FIRE
BRIGADE

6

A few years ago I read a wonderful analogy by a gentleman called James Chestnut which explained the difference between medical and alternative therapies and when you need use them. It is the best analogy I have heard and the easiest to understand, so I am using it here and adding to it slightly (thank you James). Like my Gold Fish Bowl analogy, it is simple but not designed to treat you like an idiot – so just go with it.

If your house is on fire, who do you call? Yes, the fire brigade. What tools do they carry to do their work? Hoses and axes. In order to save your house, they axe down the doors and pump powerful jets of water into every corner of the burning house. Their aim is to stop the fire *before* your house dies a horrible death. That is their only aim. They do not care what damage is done in order to meet this objective and nor should they. The doors get smashed in, windows broken and everything is ruined either by the fire itself or by the water they have used. They even hose areas where there is no fire to stop the spread. They do their job. Although the inside of the house is in extremely bad shape – the windows out and doors axed to bits, plaster off the walls and so on – your house has survived. You are extremely grateful. It could have been a great deal worse, but you are also upset, because your house is now in extremely bad condition.

Now, in order to repair the house, who do you call? Carpenters, plumbers, decorators, plasterers, locksmiths and glaziers. You would never, ever, under any circumstances call the fire brigade to fix your house up. Why? Because they don't have the correct tools for the job! They have hoses and axes, and their skills are to blast water onto to fire and to do whatever is needed to get into the building and to stop the fire spreading.

They are not trained to plaster or decorate, nor do they have the tools to do so.

As you have probably gathered, the fire brigade represents the emergency medical services, and the builders and repairers represent the correct nutrients, rest and exercise required for healing and optimum health.

Yes, we need intervention when it comes to medical emergencies, and there will *always* be a need for the 'fire-brigade' to come in and do whatever they can to save the burning building. The water and axes are of course toxic, if you will, to a non-burning house and would, if used in the way they are used when a house is burning, cause great damage to that house that isn't burning. However, if the house is burning down, they are the *only* tools that can save it. The same goes for some diseases; medical drugs and emergency procedures are the *only* way to go. In some cases, the body is in such a state of disrepair and is essentially, for the sake of this analogy, burning to death, that it needs the medical equivalent of the fire brigade.

And let's not lose perspective here either. Some of the breakthroughs in medical science in the 21st century, when it comes to emergency treatment and keeping people alive, are nothing short of remarkable – truly breath-taking in fact. Something that now seems as normal as laser eye surgery is off-the-scale life changing for all those who have it done. What the medical profession does to save lives in A & E every single day is beyond anything my brain can fathom; it is truly remarkable and nothing in nature can replace what these incredible people do. The medical profession saves hundreds of thousands of lives on a daily basis by using expert emergency intervention. Car accidents, fractures, bone breaks, heart attacks, strokes, cancers (depending on their stage) are just some of the examples where medical emergency intervention is often very necessary.

If your house is on fire
you need the Emergency Service.
IF IT'S NOT – YOU DON'T!

The problem is that BIG PHARMA have a way with words, or rather with 'scientific research' and it's often enough to convince us to take their particular drug 'just in case'. Adding to James Chestnut's 'fire brigade' analogy, I wish to extend it slightly to illustrate just how easily BIG PHARMA & CO can use 'science' to put fear into you and to convince you the only way forward is to take their drug every day for life. There's science fact and then there's …

SCIENCE FICTION

FICTION

The Art Of

Misdirection

1

Imagine I'm in the business of selling hoses and water. I get a nice amount of profit by selling you the hose initially, but the real money is in the water. I get a kick-back from all the water you use, so it's in my interest to make sure you use as much of it as possible on a daily basis. So how exactly am I going to not only sell you the hose but also convince you that you need to use a certain amount of water every day? How am I going to achieve this when, up until now, you've managed perfectly well without the hose or the water?

The answer is simple: FEAR. All I need to do is create enough fear and you'll buy a hose and start using the water in no time. How do I create this fear? Good-ole scientific research, and this is where the misdirection comes in.

In the village where you live, due to the incredibly hot weather, a few houses burn down each year. It is a growing problem and one you know that your house may be at risk of. Having said that, out of hundreds of thousands of houses, only two or three ever 'die', if you will, of house fire. The risk is incredibly low and not something you ever really think or worry about. This is where I come in. I need to you think and, specifically, I need you to worry. Worry causes fear and people act when fearful.

Imagine I conduct an experiment in your village to prove that if you use my method there is a 100 per cent chance your house will never burn to the ground. In other words I can 'cure' it of 'death by house fire' and remove all if the risk. Here's what I do. The village has two sides to it and a river flows through the middle. I take one side only for my research. My job is to prevent the houses dying of house fire, nothing more and nothing less. On the study group side I hose the outside and inside of the houses twice a day every day. I blast every nook and cranny, inside and out.

At the end of the year-long study the results are in. On the side where the houses weren't treated there were indeed some house deaths caused by fire. In fact it was a particularly bad year and four houses died of fire. However, on the other side of the river, none of the houses which had been treated with my method died of house fire.

I write up my paper and show conclusive 'proof' that my approach prevents house-fire deaths. However, what it doesn't report – and you can see where this is going – are any of the houses that died of something other than house fire. Virtually all the houses that have died in the study group have either died of wet rot, or they've crumbled, or they're very sick and in disrepair, because they've had water blasted onto and into every part of the building for a year. However, my research paper doesn't have to report that a house died of anything other than house fire. I was there to 'prove' that, by following my method, you could effectively prevent all house-fire deaths. The fact that many more in the study group died of other things is neither here nor there; my report doesn't have to show this. It only has to show how many died of house fire.

Now, clearly anyone in their right mind would start blasting their walls, inside and out, every day with massive jets of water to prevent their house dying of house fire. Of course, they would intuitively know that this treatment would ultimately cause more problems than it solves. However, drugs and human disease are different and it's extremely easy for BIG PHARMA to 'prove' a drug can prevent this or that by simply applying a little misdirection and fear, and they do it in spades! Unlike the hose and water analogy, when a person with a medical background starts reeling off supposedly convincing research data and begins to tell you that you have an X per cent chance of this or that happening to you unless you start to take this pill every day for life, trust me, you'll take the pill.

The art of misdirection within the 'science-based' medical drug field is enough to make Derren (never call him Darren) Brown look like an amateur. If they are doing trials on a drug and 100 trials, say, show serious adverse side effects and two show improvements, they simply discard the 100 which show problems and write up the results reporting just the two trials that showed positive results. David Copperfield has nothing on these guys, and it's why you will hear time and time again that a drug once hailed as a wonder drug has been taken off the market owing to adverse side-effects which didn't come to light when first approved by people such as the MHRA in the UK or the FDA in the USA:

As I keep repeating and repeating, and as I really, really, really don't wish anyone to misunderstand anything I am saying in this book:

AT TIMES WE NEED MEDICAL DRUGS, AND YOU SHOULD ALWAYS CONSULT YOUR DOCTOR BEFORE DOING A PROGRAMME OF THIS NATURE OR BEFORE THINKING ABOUT COMING OFF ANY MEDICAL DRUGS

Equally:

THERE IS A MASSIVE OVERUSE OF MEDICAL DRUGS FOR CONDITIONS WHICH COULD BE TREATED BY THE BODY'S NATURAL HEALING PROCESS, IF GIVEN THE RIGHT TOOLS AND ENVIRONMENT TO DO SO

This is why so many seemingly 'different' conditions improve massively with exactly the same *Super Juice Me! 28-Day Plan*. It is known that most common conditions and diseases are caused by inflammation and it is also known that virtually all fruits and vegetables are natural anti-inflammatories. The *Super Juice Me!* plan works because it removes all inflammatory foods and drinks and replaces them with pure anti-inflammatory foods (in liquid form to be precise). Doesn't it stand to common-sense reason that many conditions would improve with such an approach?

The proof of the pudding is of course in the eating – well, in this case, in not eating it – and you shouldn't knock it till you've tried it. The only reason I am writing all of this before presenting you with the plan itself is to put your mind at rest that what you are about embark on is not in anyway dangerous or harmful. I have written about BIG PHARMA,

THE GOLDFISH BOWL, THE FIRE BRIGADE and so on to illustrate what is happening so that you don't simply buy into what someone tells you or advises simply because they are wearing a white coat and have the appropriate certificates to match. Equally, I am saying don't just buy into what I'm saying either. It's good to be healthily sceptical. Take what makes sense to you and use it. And don't finally judge until you've tried it on for size.

We need to remember, though, that medical research has been wrong on many occasions. I believe that doing things like removing sections of a child's stomach to combat his or her obesity issue, or giving everyone over the age of 40 a statin just in case they get heart disease, is not the most intelligent way to go about things. I have also tried to give as many examples as this small book would allow of people who have done the *Super Juice Me! 28-Day Juice Challenge* and experienced incredible changes to a whole host of different diseases. I have done this to give you the confidence to at least do the 28-Day *Super Juice Me! Challenge*.

Even as we speak, there are so many results coming in on a daily basis that I will be producing a free download of *Super Juice Me!* results to help inspire others. There really are that many! You can dismiss one or two as anecdotal but, as I said at the beginning, when you start getting thousands all saying the same thing, it's time to sit up and pay attention – even if it goes against everything you thought was true before. It was always believed, for example, that anyone with type 2 diabetes shouldn't juice because it could cause them to have sugar spikes, and all the doctors I ever spoke to when starting this said, 'Do not recommend this for people with diabetes'. Yet I have had many people with diabetes do this programme and either improve or turn their condition around completely; a few examples are in the book. This goes against the old school of thought, but just because it's against what was or is still believed to be true in many circles doesn't actually make it false or wrong.

ALL JUICE SCEPTICS VERY WELCOME

The number of juice sceptics I get is ever increasing. What I have found though is that these are people who have either never actually tried it or who only did a day or two and then threw in the towel. I have had TV doctors openly pooh-pooh on live TV what I am doing, and dieticians in the press openly saying how 'dangerous' my programmes are. It is very easy to criticize something one has not tried personally. If they spent as much time actually speaking to the people who have been 'Super Juiced' and analysing their results as they do criticizing from afar, maybe they'd change their minds and maybe, just maybe, they might even recommend it as an alternative to drugs-based therapy. Maybe, just maybe, they'd recommend it over extremely costly bariatric surgery, and maybe, just maybe, it would go some way to ending the 'pill for every ill and ill for every pill' culture that is plaguing most of the western world today.

There is a long way to go before that happens, but with each new *Super Juice Me!* story, with each ailment or disease that improves through this approach, the greater the chance we have of the right people paying attention and the greater the chance we have of getting 'juice therapy' as a genuine and credible treatment for various health conditions. You never know, we may even see juicing in hospitals one day – not that the usual microwave food isn't appealing of course! (Gordon Ramsay, if you ever read this, let's team up and really make a difference by getting some decent nutrition into hospitals.) One day 'juicing in hospitals' might already be a reality. We can only hope.

What's quite exciting is that you can play a part in that change. All you have to do is to jump on the juice wagon, get yourself Super Juiced! and send us your results.

SO ARE YOU UP FOR *THE SUPER JUICE ME!* 28-DAY JUICE CHALLENGE?

Most people who buy books of this nature, never actually follow through on them. When 'clicking to basket' or downloading they are convinced that 'this is it' and 'this time' they will do what it takes to stops talking and start doing. However, after 15 years of doing this I have come to one realization: people are very good at buying books, but reading them and actually acting upon them is another thing. It is estimated that over 70 per cent of self-help books are left unread. As an example, in the UK we buy more cookery books and watch more cookery shows than any other European nation, and yet we buy twice as many takeaways, a statistic which illustrates our amazing ability to buy the books, watch the shows, but never actually follow what's in them.

The fact you are reading this sentence some 115 pages into the book tells me that you just may be one of the exceptions to the rule. It tells me you might actually take up the *Super Juice Me! 28-Day Juice Challenge* and do whatever it takes to complete it and reap the truly incredible rewards which lie at the end. In fact, if I could somehow transport you 28 days into the future and have you experience for just five minutes how you will look and how incredible you will feel at the end of the challenge, you'd start tomorrow morning! I know you should undersell and over deliver, but having personally done this challenge a couple of times, it's hard to undersell it. You only have to read all the testimonials scattered throughout the whole book to know what is potentially in store for you.

However, there is one final obstacle that can prevent you from ever starting and/or finishing the challenge. It's the one thing that, in my opinion, prevents more people from getting the body and health they ultimately crave than any other single factor. I am a strong believer in the adage you cannot get into the right frame of body without first getting into the right frame of mind. To that end, if you want true success and not a fridge full of mouldy fruit and veg, as your best intentions go out the window a few days in, it's time to…

DITCH THE EXCUSES!

8

I have been doing this now for over 15 years and I have come to one conclusion:

THE ONLY THINGS PREVENTING ANYONE FROM GETTING THE BODY AND HEALTH THEY CRAVE ARE EXCUSES!

And I've heard them all. Not only have I heard them all, I've also worn the excuse tee shirt many times in my life. I believe we're all guilty of this on many occasions, and we unfortunately now live in a world that laps this crap up. It seems we need to over analyse the arse out of everything, especially when searching for good enough reasons to justify why we cannot lose weight and get healthy. We now live in in the world of blame, and society in general not only allows it, but feeds it at every opportunity. We blame our past, our lack of time, our lack of money, our metabolism, our being 'big boned'. We blame the people around us; we blame other people who have failed; we even blame the weather! In short:

We blame everyone and everything for why we can't put the donut down and get ourselves up ...

... everything apart from us that is!

It appears most of us have an arsenal of excuses in our weaponry, and we're ready to use them at any sign that we might actually be thinking of making a change. All of our excuses sound, on the surface, perfectly plausible and valid, not only to ourselves, but more importantly, to everyone else around us. All of them are designed to justify why we either fail to act at all or give up early on a goal or challenge. One thing is for sure, it is never really our fault, but merely the fact we are victims of circumstances out of our control. It's all part of what I describe as the, 'YES BUT...' world, a world in which the vast majority of people reside, and a world in which society allows people to comfortably – or to be more accurate on a physical front, *uncomfortably* – sit. The 'YES BUT...' world is one in which, if someone comes up with a perfectly good counter-argument for whatever excuse a person has given and provides them with a way they could in fact change, boom, they immediately come back with a 'YES BUT...'

It's irrelevant how they finish this sentence; it's all essentially BS anyway, designed with only one objective: to justify their failure to get off their arse to do something about their situation. Trust me, find someone who is overweight and you'll find a, 'YES BUT...' sentence coming out of their mouth before you can say 'Hobnobs'! This may sound harsh, but I know this because I was overweight for years and all I ever did was essentially 'YES BUT...' my way to having larger breasts than the average glamour model. My 'YES BUT ...' sentences, or excuses as they actually were, were designed to suit whatever sounded plausible and justifiable at the time, not only to other people but also to myself. They were all designed to justify my current behaviour and failures. It's far easier to blame than it is to take a cold hard look at ourselves, and it's far easier to tear down than it is to build.

YOUR HEALTH IS <u>YOUR</u> RESPONSIBILITY

The bottom line is this: the buck stops with you and you alone. You can blame everyone and everything for as long as you like, but until you take personal responsibility and just crack on with it, your situation will never get any better. In fact, it can only get worse.

In the movie, *The Shawshank Redemption* there's one main theme that runs throughout which works well here:

GET BUSY LIVING OR GET BUSY DYING

And that's about the strength of it. Every day we wake up with that choice. We can either get busy living or we can get busy dying; we either do something to grow or we slowly wilt; we either move forward or we go backwards. Like all animals on earth, we don't have the luxury of simply staying where we are. Fight-or-flight is built within all of us, and if a wild animal just sat around it wouldn't survive for very long. This is why a person's health and weight situation just gets worse when they do nothing about it. It's why we now have the mind-blowing situation where there are not just one or two, but *thousands* of people on the planet who weigh more than 500lbs! It's also why we now live in a world where two out of three of us will die from either cancer or heart disease and where the majority of people in western society are overweight or obese.

The sad truth is that most of these lifestyle diseases are simply caused by what we put into our mouths, which means that we have much more control than we think. And when it comes to being overweight or obese, the brutal truth is that 100 per cent of it is caused by what we put into our mouths.

DO YOU WANT THE TRUTH?
YOU CAN'T HANDLE THE TRUTH!

No doubt some people reading this page will now be shouting their, 'YES BUT, JASON…' quite loudly at this point. 'YES BUT, JASON… I've got a slow metabolism and it's not my fault'; or maybe, 'YES BUT, JASON… I've got an issue with my thyroid and I can't lose weight'; or 'YES BUT, JASON… you just don't understand'. I honestly don't care what, 'YES BUT, JASON…' a person comes up with, and as harsh as this may sound, they're all

TOTAL BS!

The only 'YES BUT JASON...' I'll buy into is when a person takes medical steroid drugs as prescribed for severe asthma, for example. Then it's possible to balloon up like crazy through no fault of the individual. Other than that, there isn't an overweight person on earth who can't lose weight, especially doing this *Super Juice Me! 28-Day Juice Challenge*. I will say it again and again, the cold hard truth is this: the only thing preventing you from getting the better health and better body you crave is your big fat EXCUSES. Drop them and you drop the weight, it's that simple. I hear so many people in this area saying, 'YES BUT... I've tried every diet under the sun and nothing works'. RUBBISH! What they mean is that they went out one Sunday, bought some fruit and veg, made a declaration to the world that 'this is it' and 'as from Monday' they're going to change their diet once and for all, only to bring out the big-gun excuses by Thursday as they watch the mouldy fruit and veg making their own way out of the fridge!

How do I know? Because I did this over and over again, week after week, year after year. Every Monday was going to be the day I changed, and every Wednesday or Thursday of that same week out came the 'BUTS', and I was back to square one. Actually I wasn't even back to square one, I was in a worse position because I just binged like crazy, sub-consciously trying to make up for the 'food' I felt I had missed out on. There has to be a point where you say, 'Enough is enough', you drop the excuses, and start. Not only start, but also finish what you started!

The fact is the *Super Juice Me! 28-Day Challenge* has been shown to work time and time again. You only have to flick to the centre pages to see that. The question isn't whether

'IT' works; it is, rather, whether you are going to do 'IT'. In other words, are you going to do the work? That means not reaching day six and coming up with some crap excuse as to why you need to reach for a cream bun. I'm talking about actually doing it and being *fully* committed. I am only saying all of this and seeming harsh because I know just how amazing you're going to feel if you do this and how much it will 'reset' your mind and taste buds. I know how good this is and I want to do everything within my power to make sure you complete the *full Super Juice Me! 28-Day Challenge*. I want to make sure you don't just start it and then bail out!

As I mentioned, if I could transport you to the end of the 28 days right now and show you exactly how you will look and feel, you'd not only start tomorrow, but you'd also love the process, and nothing could stop you. In fact you'd be leaping up and down with excitement. As crazy or as unbelievable as it may sound now, it doesn't matter how 'addicted' you are to junk, do this plan and by the time you finish you'll be craving salads!

Don't believe me? Try it. What's the worst that can happen? This isn't just about the 28 days, it's how it totally 'resets' your mind and body and how it triggers a natural desire for natural food. Read the very first testimonial in this book, the one I had to 'hold the front page' for. The *Super Juice Me!* plan reset his mind so much he even kicked his addiction to drugs like cocaine, so sugar doesn't stand a chance!

No matter how daunting the thought of living on nothing but juices for 28 days may seem now, there is always a way *if* you're committed. And I guess the million-dollar question is this: are you truly committed? Are you willing to do *whatever it takes* to complete the *Super Juice Me! 28-Day Challenge*? Are you willing to stay focused for 28 days and reap the rewards?

What I have learnt over the years and a truth I keep repeating in my all of my books is this:

THE MORE 'BUTS' YOU COME UP WITH THE BIGGER BUTT YOU'LL END UP WITH!

I don't care how busy you are, how much you've got on, what's happening in your life, if you really want to make it happen – there is always a way.

> We just did my husband's measurements on day 28. He has lost a whopping 3" around his chest, 5" off his waist and 2" off his hips, I am so impressed, he stuck it through to the end and is now really "on it" to continue with healthy choices and still juicing within that. We are both feeling so much stronger in all sorts of ways and on many levels. Thank you, Jason Vale Juice Master, for this so easy to follow programme, for me it has been great not having to think about anything other than getting the shopping in, as we are both super busy at the moment, working stupid hours 7 days a week. In fact today we are finally having a day off! It just proves that there are no "I'm too busy" excuses to not do the programme, it was all a matter of, as Jason says, "What do we need to do to make this happen". Thanks once again.
>
> **C. Des-Rivieres**

I appreciate that it's never going to seem the right time, and there will be something coming up in a 28-day period – a dinner party, someone's birthday and so on – but that will always be the case. There are only 12 months in a year, so inevitably there will a few social hurdles to jump during the challenge. However, if I offered you £1 million to make it happen you would do it!

Your health is the most valuable asset you will ever have, it is your *everything*, and it is the only place where true wealth ever lives. After all, would you rather be a multi-millionaire lying in bed on a drip, or skint and riding a surfboard? Would you rather be minted and waddling along a beach in glorious sunshine, barely able to breathe and having to cover up your body because you don't want anyone to see it, or would you rather not know where your next pay cheque is coming from but be able to run freely along a beach in your swimming gear? The truth is, you can have all the money in the world, but if don't have the pure energy and vibrant health to do what you want in life, you are ultimately very poor.

Over the years I have known many millionaires and some billionaires, and they are the first to realise you cannot buy health, you can only earn it. Yes, you can buy plastic surgery to alter your external appearance and pay to get some fat sucked out of you, but that doesn't make you healthy. It doesn't build your immune system to help fight disease, nor does it give you pure energy or help you to be mentally razor sharp. All it does is to change some external features of your body – often making people look worse than before they started. Is it me, or do a lot of people in LA now resemble a duck?

STOP 'HOPING' AND DECIDE!

If you want *real* and permanent change in this area of your life, you need to make a *real* decision. The word 'decision' comes from the Latin decidere, which literally means 'to cut off from' – to cut off from any other possibility. A few of the dictionary's definitions for 'decide' are:

- **To make a final choice or judgement about**
- **To select a course of action**
- **To bring to a definitive end**
- **To induce to come to a choice**

If you really want to do *Super Juice Me! 28-Day Challenge*, then decide to do it – truly decide. To decide is not to hope, it is to know. It is to 'cut off from any other possibility'. It is to 'make a final judgement and select a course of action'. To decide is to have absolute certainty. You already have a course of action laid out in this book; all you need to do now is to decide to follow it. Don't hope you'll complete it, or start saying you *would* BUT…, or you *should* BUT…, or you *could* BUT…, etc. *Know for certain* you're going to follow it. The truth is that you can *hope, would, should, could* all over yourself, and nothing will ever change. To make a true decision is extremely powerful and changes your life's course.

The reason that so many people don't do something about their health and weight is because they focus on what they perceive to be the 'cost' of making the changes, without ever looking at what is often the truly horrific costs of *not* making the changes. We all say, 'Without our health we've got nothing', but just saying it whilst shoving a muffin into your mouth and never getting up off your arse does nothing to change your situation. So many people talk a great game, but that's all they do – talk. There are two kinds of people in this world: those who *talk* about making a change, and those who finally stop talking and take *action*. Whenever I hear anyone saying, 'Oh, I'm *thinking* about starting my own business', or 'Oh I'm *thinking* about writing a book', or 'I'm *thinking* about doing the *Super Juice Me! 28-Day Juice Challenge*', I very rarely take any notice of what they are saying. I tend to nod and say, 'That's good'. But I'm not engaged at all, and I don't believe a word of it. However, tell me you're actually doing it, tell me you're two chapters into writing your book, or that you've signed a lease for your new business premises, or you're on day seven of the *Super Juice Me!* plan, then I'm all ears!

Talk is very cheap and talk can be very, very costly. The effort it requires to make a decision, take action and follow through on your goal is nothing compared to the effort and subsequent pain a person suffers daily, now as well as later in life by *not* taking action, especially when it comes to this area of your life.

We seem to totally dismiss the daily nightmare of being overweight and ill and instead focus on the apparent effort and pain it would take to get slim and well. We very wrongly conclude that doing nothing is much less effort and less painful than doing something about our health and weight situation. We also wrongly feel that we'd making tremendous sacrifices by changing what we eat, completely ignoring, of course, the many, many sacrifices we have to make daily *because* of the crap we eat. We don't ever focus on this side of life, but we blindly, *daily*, make huge sacrifices as a direct result of the rubbish going into our body. We sacrifice our health, our energy, our peace of mind, our self-respect, our courage, our confidence, and our freedom to move every day the way we'd love to. We sacrifice what we want to wear or where we feel comfortable on holiday. We sacrifice our time, our money and, ultimately, the very quality and length of our one-and-only life on this planet.

Just think just how much your current weight and state of health is genuinely costing you. Think about how long you spend trying on different clothes and getting totally down and peed-off because nothing seems to look good or fit. Think now about how much just this one aspect affects your life. Think what not feeling good about yourself really costs you, every single day. Think about how your health may be preventing you from doing what you really want to do and about how much that is costing you every single day. You are making all of these sacrifices – and more – every single day. Each day is getting worse than the previous one, and all for what? What do you really get out of your current diet and lack of exercise that's worth paying this price for? What, in real terms, would you actually be giving up? A bit of refined fat, salt and sugar that *ultimately* make you feel like crap anyway. Think about what you are giving up every day by not making the change.

FROM 'DIET MENTALITY' TO 'FREEDOM MENTALITY'

I believe this is where everyone gets it so, so, wrong when 'going on a diet' of any kind. Even before you start you're under the false belief that you'll be making huge sacrifices and, as a consequence, you end up diving straight into what I call a 'diet mentality'. It is not usually the food on the diet that's the problem, but rather the diet mentality a person adopts and puts themselves through, when on that diet.

When you have a diet mentality you take a deep breath, clench your fists, and put yourself into a constant state of mental deprivation. You constantly focus on what you feel you can't have, rather than on what you have the opportunity to have. It's where you effectively force yourself into what can only be described as a self-imposed mental tantrum and spend your day moping around for the foods and drinks you feel you can't have. I say, '*feel* you can't have', because nothing is actually stopping you from having whatever you like at any time, even during the 28-Day juice challenge. You can physically go to the shop, pick up any food and just it eat it.

But the point is that you don't want to! You *want* to stop the crap, you *want* to feel amazing, you *want* to wear whatever you like, you *want* great health, you want more energy. You don't want to feel like you do now, and you don't want to fail! So why put yourself into a self-imposed mental bind every day? That's what people on diets do, and they wonder why they find it hard to diet and ultimately fail.

The craziest thing is that what you'd effectively be doing if you went down the 'diet mentality' route is that you'd be moping around for certain foods and drinks you actually hope you won't have. Seriously, think about that for a moment, let that sink in, and it should enable you to realize why so many people fail on diets of any kind. How insane would that be, getting upset or angry because you don't have certain foods or drinks that you really hope you won't have?

A few years ago at one of my juice retreats this guy pulled me to one side on day three and said, 'I WANT SOME FOOD!' He wasn't a happy camper. He explained how he was a very successful businessman and if he wanted food he would just have some. He didn't want to be a 'prisoner'. The retreat at the time was up a mountain in the middle of nowhere. The nearest shop was down the mountain, about 10km away.

To his surprise, I didn't respond with a 'Well, you can't'. I simply said, 'Sure, what do you want?' I said I had a moped and was shooting down the mountain myself, as I needed to get some stationery for the retreat, and he was welcome to join me on the back. I asked what kind of food did he want, and explained they served just about everything down there, from steak and chips, burgers and fries, to the most indulgent chocolate cake he could imagine.

He then said, 'No, I don't want to. I want to finish this. I just really want some food.' I said, 'If you really want some, let's go!' To which, he replied, 'NO I DON'T WANT TO.' I said, 'SO SHUT UP, THEN!'

Now, before he had a chance to punch me for being so

rude, I explained what I meant by my 'shut up!' comment, and he immediately got it. Diet mentality is nothing more than a psychological tug-of-war. One side says, 'I want'; the other says, 'I can't'. This creates feelings of deprivation and sacrifice, and it's this tug-of-war people go through on diets that leads to their ultimate downfall.

My aim here is to make the *Super Juice Me!* challenge as easy as possible for you. I will tell you now that it all comes down to what you say to yourself every day, nothing more than that. I know that sounds simple, but it is simple if you go about it the right way. You will be getting more than enough genuine nutrition, so any thoughts of starving or 'I need more fuel' are completely unfounded. The *only thing* that can make it hard for you is adopting the diet mentality and telling yourself all day long that you *can't* have this or *can't* have that. The truth is that you can have what the bloody hell you want, but you don't want it. That's the point! If you ever feel this tug of war rearing its ugly head, you can do one of two things: you can either have 'it' (whatever food or drink that represents to you) and shut up; or you can do without 'it' and shut up. BUT SHUT UP! You need to understand that it's only the moping for something you hope you won't have that can possibly cause you any problems at all. You simply need to shift from a 'I want it but can't have it' mind-set to a 'I *can* have it but don't want it' mind-set. You need to shift from diet mentality to freedom mentality. You are *choosing* to have fresh juice for a month for all of the reasons that lead you to be reading this page. You are choosing to not have the crap. We live in a world of abundance and you *can* have anything at any time, but you are *choosing* not to.

FREE AND EASY

A freedom mentality is just that: one in which you feel free. You are freeing yourself from so many things, not just from excess weight and ill health, but also from the slavery and control of these highly processed and addictive foods. You will soon be free to wear what you want, go where you want and live your life the way you want. This should be an exciting venture, not one of doom or gloom. You are doing something about the most valuable commodity you will ever own – your body and health. There is great power in your freedom mentality. It's where you can have anyone cooking around you or eating anything around you and know you have the freedom *not to have* to have the food that's being cooked or eaten. This is the main problem with food addiction: all freedom of genuine choice has been removed.

YOU CANNOT HAVE FREEDOM OF GENUINE CHOICE WITHOUT THE FREEDOM TO REFUSE

People often say it's their choice to eat crap, but you cannot have freedom of genuine choice without also having the freedom to refuse. I love bananas; it is my genuine choice to eat them. I know it is my genuine choice, because I have the genuine freedom to refuse them too. If my doctor had told me that my banana eating was causing my obesity, skin problems, asthma, hay fever and over-all ill health, do you honestly think I'd have any issues stopping my intake? Do you think that because I love the taste so much I wouldn't be able to stop? Of course not? Why? Because bananas are a natural food, not a drug-like food. They don't create the fear that I wouldn't be able to enjoy or cope with my life the same way without them! Not only would I have not a jot of an issue stopping bananas if they were the thing causing my illnesses and obesity, but I'd be elated because I now had the answer. I would be doing cartwheels, because I would know the cause of my problems. All I'd have to do would be to stop eating bananas and I'd be slim and well. Do you think I'd ever envy anyone eating a banana? The answer is no, because I *can* have one whenever I want. I just would never want.

This is why you should be starting this challenge with a feeling of excitement, *knowing* – not hoping – that you'll feel like a new person in just 28 days, *knowing* that you'll reset your body and taste buds in just 28 days to give you ultimate control over what you eat in the future. This is why I never understand anyone starting this challenge with a feeling of dread. The real challenge would be to live your life without doing anything to help your situation.

And while we're here, let's put this 'challenge' into total perspective. All you are doing is living on freshly extracted juices and smoothies for 28 days; you're not swimming the channel or climbing Mount Everest. I'm not underplaying what you'll be doing, but I'm writing this page having just come out of the most inspirational one-hour talk I have ever had the good fortune to attend, given by a guy called John Maclean. If you hear this man's story, then living on nothing but juice for 28 days would be put into total perspective and wouldn't even register as a 'challenge'.

THE TRUCK MOMENT

There is no way I can do this incredible man's story justice here; we don't have time. But I'll give you the highlights. If you get the chance, you have to read his book. In fact I challenge you to read his book before you start this. If you do read his book, the *Super Juice Me! 28-Day Challenge* will become one of the easiest things you will ever do. Perspective is everything.

In 1988 John Maclean had what he describes as a 'truck moment'. He was training for a triathlon when he was knocked off his bike by an eight-tonne truck, a truck moment which left him a paraplegic. He still had use of his upper body but had no movement from the waist down. Now, for most people this would have been a good enough reason to no longer do the triathlon. But John isn't 'most people'; he epitomizes what true commitment and spirit are made of. He also demonstrates what a 'no excuses' attitude really looks like. To cut a very powerful and long story short, he not only completed a triathlon in 1994, but a year later he became the first paraplegic to complete the Ironman World Championship in Hawaii.

If you don't know what an Ironman triathlon is, let me tell you. First you swim for 2.4 miles (3.86km); then you get on a bike and cycle for 112 miles (180.25 km); you then finish things off with a marathon (26.2 miles or 42.2km). That's a marathon after you've already swum 2.4 miles and cycled 112 miles! To do this as an able-bodied person is one of the hardest tests of endurance anyone can ever go through; to do this as a paraplegic takes a kind of focus and spirit that few are ever willing to give. John dropped just short of the bike 'cut-off time' for able-bodied athletes and knew this before even starting the marathon leg of the race. It took everything he had to cross the finish line.

Just finishing the Ironman as a paraplegic is mind-blowing enough, but he completed it the following year too, just narrowly missing the cut off time once again, this time due to a flat tyre! He was determined to make all the cut-off times, so he came back the following year and smashed them! John not only finished within the able-bodied cut-off times, but he beat a third of the field and became the first ever wheelchair category winner.

In 1998 a friend of his asked if he'd like to go for a 'little swim'. That swim was the English Channel. What I didn't know until listening to John's talk was that more people have successfully climbed Mount Everest than have swum the English Channel. In his talk he explained just how genuinely challenging swimming the English Channel is, especially if you can only use your arms! On his first attempt he was half way across when two-metre swells forced him to stop. Most people would have called it a day, but John doesn't have a 'most people' mentality and two weeks later he was on the shores of England to try again. Twelve hours and fifty-five minutes after setting out he was in France.

John's story goes way beyond what I've briefly outlined here, and I urge you to read his books, *Sucking The Marrow Out Of Life: The John Maclean Story* and *Full Circle: One Life, Many Lessons*. If you get a chance to see him speak live it will blow your mind. The only reason I have added a little of his story here is to put the *Super Juice Me! Challenge* into total perspective and to show you what can be achieved by dropping all excuses and doing whatever it takes to succeed.

After his truck moment John could have spent the rest of his life doing nothing and blaming the truck driver for his not having gone on to achieve anything. Instead he decided to 'Get Busy Living'. John lives by the mantra 'ONLY POSSIBILITIES': he sees only what is possible in a situation and refuses to live by a victim mentality.

We all have 'truck moments' to various degrees. You either become a victim of them or you use them to make you stronger and to make a difference. We all have a story too. It's what you do with that story that counts. You can be a victim of your story, telling it over and over again to anyone who will listen so that you can bask in their sympathy and justify why you don't change, or you can use your story to move you forward. It's not your *story* that defines you, it's *what you do* with your story that defines you. What we are truly capable of and what we are willing to do are two very different things. One thing is for sure, you can continue to blame everyone and everything for your current state of weight and health; you can 'But it's different for me because… 'your way through the rest of your life, but you'll regret it.

Trust me, you don't want to arrive in a few years saying, 'If only I'd done something then'. You won't just regret it in the long run either; you'll regret it every single day you have to live with obesity and ill health. You'll regret it every time you get dressed, every time you want to sunbathe in public. You'll regret it every time you want to play with your kids but are too tired. You'll regret it day in and day out, and you'll really, really regret it if one day you're hit by a health 'truck moment' there's no coming back from.

Prevention is much easier than cure. What you do now really does make a huge difference to your future. I don't know you personally and I don't know your situation, but I do know that if this book helps just one person reading it to take up the challenge and change the course of their health it will have been well worth it. I know some of you who are reading this simply need to lose a few pounds and might be thinking this is all too heavy and repetitive and doesn't really affect you. Please don't kid yourself. What you put into your system now will affect you in your future. I smoked three packets of cigarettes a day, drank shed-loads of alcohol and ate no plant food whatsoever for years on end. Will I have to pay a price for this later on? I don't know. Probably. Only the future will tell us that, but it will be nowhere near the price I'd be paying right now if I hadn't made the change. I honestly don't believe I'd be here today if I hadn't decided to stop most of the rubbish, quit smoking and get more plant food inside my system. We don't have a crystal ball, but you don't need to be Mystic Meg to realize that if we don't move our bodies enough and get the right nutrition on board we will, in one way or another, pay the price. And the biggest point I have been trying to get across in this chapter is that you are already paying the price to some degree or another.

THE COST OF NOT CHANGING TOTALLY DWARFS THE COST OF JUST DOING IT!

It's only 28 days and what's the worst that can happen? You get more fruit and veg inside you than you've had in a long time, you drop some weight and feel alive. That really is the worst that can happen, despite what some around you may say while you're it. Which brings me onto the final warning:

WATCH OUT FOR OTHER PEOPLE. THEY WON'T ALWAYS BE HAPPY ABOUT YOU GETTING THINNER AND HEALTHIER!

You'd think this is the one area where you'd get more support from friends and family than any other, but don't you believe it. Everyone wants to give the impression of support, and some will of course be genuine, but many people will be fearful of your change. Look at it this way, if you live next door to a friend and both of your houses look pretty much same, there's no issue. However, if you decide to improve your house and make it look amazing inside and out, then you may start to experience a few problems with the neighbours. What you have inadvertently done by making improvements to your house is to highlight how much worse their houses now look. There are just a couple of ways of solving this issue. They can either do what it takes to improve their own houses and make them look better, or they can simply blow yours up! Unfortunately many choose the latter and the second you start to make a change they will do what they can to sabotage it. When it comes to this particular programme – 28 days of *only* juice – they will try to freak you out by telling you that it's 'unhealthy' or 'dangerous'.

What I find odd is the same people never felt the same urge to express these same points when you were eating rubbish and suffering from overweight and various ills. It really is an odd world we live in. Tell someone you're cutting out all the rubbish and having only plant food for a while and they freak out and think it's dangerous; but tell them you've decided to f**k healthy eating and you're having a blow out and will be getting as drunk as a skunk, and not a peep! You'll hear people say, 'How are you going to live on nothing but juice? That's stupid', yet they don't ask the questions of someone who eats nothing but potato chips, chocolate, burgers, fries, and drinks shed-loads of alcohol and 'energy' drinks.

The point I am making is this: no one minds you getting slim and healthy, *providing you are miserable*! If you're happy about it and not struggling the way people usually do on any diet (due to having a diet mentality), they'll hate you. However, if you are moaning every day, saying how hard it is and 'white knuckle riding it', as it were, they'll know there's a good chance you'll bail before you're house is fully refurbished. This will give them hope. After all, if you make it, your house will look amazing, and this will simply highlight how bad their house might look. This is why they'll try many times to do what they can to stop you completing it. 'It's dangerous', 'you're mad', 'it's unhealthy', are just a few of the gambits, but most of the time it will be the 'come on, life's short, you could get run over by a bus' approach that they'll use to put the brakes on your 'house improvements'. All I am saying is, watch out for them. 'Forewarned is forearmed', as they say, and I want to cover all the bases while we are here.

The reason I use the house analogy is because I once heard a sentence that completely changed my world. It is so simple, yet had such a profound impact on my health. I included it in one of my earlier books, but since many people are being introduced to my world through this book, I want to repeat it here.

It was an 87-year-old man who was living on the streets who had perhaps the most profound impact on my health, and he will be blissfully unaware of the fact. He was featured in one of those '60 Minutes' type documentaries, with a few stories in an hour-long show. The programme was looking at the longest-lived people across the world and finding out what their secrets are. This particular Irish 87-year-old lived on the streets of London, had all his own teeth and hair, and looked the very picture of health. The interviewer asked him a very simple question: 'What's your secret?' The man quickly replied, 'I never eat junk food.'

'But you don't have a choice, surely,' the interviewer said. 'You live on the street and you can only eat what you're given.'

The 87-year-old replied that this wasn't the case at all. He helped out at the local fruit-and-veg market and they gave him free fruit and veg in return for his help. He also said a local restaurant owner gave him some lean proteins and veg at the end of the night to save it going to waste.

Then the interviewer asked a question which sums up the 'food trap' most of us are in. 'OK, I can see you're in a position to not eat junk food, but why don't you? You're 87 years of age and you've got to live a bit.' That just goes to show that most people feel you can't really 'live' unless you shove some crap into your mouth.

The old man's reply was priceless and more profound than perhaps he realized himself, and it's worth emphasizing. He simply replied,

'THE REASON I DON'T EAT JUNK FOOD IS BECAUSE UNLESS I LOOK AFTER MY BODY I'LL HAVE NOWHERE TO LIVE.'

And that me just about sums it up. Unless we look after our body, we'll have nowhere to live. Yes we'll always have somewhere to *survive*, but we'll have nowhere to truly live. Your life is only as good as how well you feel and as the 'house' that you get to live your life in. The *Super Juice Me! 28-Day Challenge* will improve your house in ways you don't even know yet, and that's why I am stupidly excited to be writing this.

Everything you need is in this book. Back-up and coaching is on the app, if you choose to get it. Preparation is key to success, so leave no stone unturned before you start. As massively overused as this saying is, it is still true: 'If you fail to prepare, you prepare to fail.'

By now you should be mentally pretty much ready to go and itching to get started. Just make sure that before you get started you do read the rest of the book. It lays out the practical side of life and covers everything so you know exactly what to do, what juicer to get, how to make every recipe, what produce to buy and so on. I feel it is also vital that you read the Q & A session at the end.

Even if you don't get to read the all of the book before you start, you must read the TOP TEN TIPS FOR JUICY SUCCESS, which is up next. You have another 28 days to read the rest, and as you won't be cooking you'll have plenty of time to read it, so no excuses.

I just want to thank you for reading the book, and I look forward to hearing your results. All the details are in the 'What's Next?' chapter later in the book. Until you reach there, enjoy the challenge and I'll see you on the other side!

TOP TEN
TIPS FOR
SUPER
JUICE ME!
SUCCESS

1. MAKE IT EASY FOR YOURSELF!

The plan has been specifically devised so that on five of the days (for most people this will be Monday – Friday), you make and consume just two different recipes per day. Although I am a massive advocate of drinking your juice within 30 minutes of it being made, I am also a realist and appreciate that many people may find it challenging to make four fresh juices per day. For this reason I have devised the plan so that the morning and evening juice of the day are the same and the mid-day and afternoon juice are also the same. This means that if time is a challenge for you, you can simply make two different recipes per day (double up each recipe) and then store the additional juice in a flask and store in the fridge until ready to consume.

I first devised this system when I was writing *5lbs in 5 Days Juice Master Detox Diet*, and the feedback was so good that it was a no-brainer to implement the same system in this 28-Day *Super Juice Me!* juice plan.

The only days when this differs slightly is at the weekends. This is because I have added some 'special guest' smoothies that could just make the difference between success and failure. The weekend *evening* juices will be one of these 'specials' (all made with fresh, raw almond milk) and are all stupidly delicious! However, your second and third juice will still be the same during the weekends, so my strong recommendation would be to follow option B below. Here are some suggestions which will help you to make it easy for yourself over the next 28 days. Take your pick!

A **Make all the juices in the morning. Store them in flasks or 'Fusion Boosters' and then drink them throughout the day. As there are usually only two *different* juices a day, it means you only have to make a double batch of the first two juices and you're done!**

If you are doing it this way, it is important to make and store the juice as quickly as possible. You are trying to prevent too much oxygen and light getting to the juice, as this can cause it to oxidise and lose vital nutrients.

B **Make and drink juice number 1 when it's 100 per cent fresh, then make and store juices 2 and 3 in advance (as above), and make your fourth, 'dinner' juice fresh at home.**

The reason for this is threefold:

1 The longer you leave any juice, even in a flask or Fusion Booster, the more the juice will lose nutrients. So, by having your first and fourth juices made fresh you are getting them 100 per cent fresh, which is always best where possible.

2 It's good for the mind to be in the kitchen making something for 'dinner', even if it's not what you usually

have. Don't underestimate just how much extra time you have in your life, especially during the evenings, when drinking juice only. If you make them all in advance it can make the evenings harder, as you might have nothing to do! Plus it means if you have a family, and there's action in the kitchen, you're not left out.

3 You only need to clean your juicer twice a day!

4 This is the option I would strongly recommend, based on 15 years of juice detox/diet experience. I feel it's a nice halfway house between 100 per cent fresh and the convenience of pre-prepared juices. Feel free to make all juices fresh at the time of drinking them. That's the ideal, but I realize it is not realistic for most.

C **If you really hate the thought of having to juice every day, you can even make all the juices on one day, store them in a bunch of flasks and freeze them. Then, simply move your juices for the next day to the fridge each night and, bingo, you're done.**

The potential issue with this is that you lose some nutrients (not huge amounts as freezing retains around 95 per cent of nutrients) and also the juice can taste a little flat. But it's an option, and I know it's easiest for some people, and it's better than not doing it at all where you clearly lose 100 per cent of the nutrients!

D **Another option that more and more people are taking up due to time pressures is to have all your juices delivered directly to your door.**

This service is available at **www.juicemasterdelivered.com.**

We juice everything in a hydraulic press and *immediately* lock in the high-quality nutrients by 'blast-freezing' them. We then deliver the juice, still frozen, direct to your door. You just take the juice out of the freezer the night before, place it in the fridge, and drink at the appropriate times the next day. You don't lose a great deal of the nutrients when you freeze the juice, and as they are made in the finest cold press juicers the quality of the juices – even once frozen – is often higher than if you made it fresh at home with a high speed juicer. If you are reading this book on its first release, the full *Super Juice Me!* juice delivery plan may not yet be available, but it's coming soon!

If you see any company claiming to be delivering 'Jason Vale' or 'Juice Master' juice plans on any site other than my own, please be aware I have not approved them. They are simply trying to make a quick buck from my name and I have seen quite a few doing it. The biggest issue I have with this is that they are using my plans and named recipes and people will think that their often very inferior product is mine. In life you often get what you pay for, and *Juice Master Delivered* isn't cheap. In fact, I would describe it as 'reassuringly expensive' (which I believe I once heard on a beer commercial).

Most people will opt to make the juices themselves and that will always be the better financial option. It will often also be the better nutritional option too. I am a massive advocate of juicing 100 per cent fresh wherever you can, and the Juice Master Delivered service is only intended for those who really don't have time to shop, prepare, juice, and clean the juicer. Time demands get ever greater for all of us. However, if you can juice at home, then put down the lazy brush and get juicing!

E *Super Juice Me!* **at Juicy Oasis in Portugal.**

This is a very expensive option, compared to either making it all yourself at home or having them all delivered through Juice Master Delivered. However, it is an option, and all details can be found on page 377. Juicy Oasis is the home of *Super Juice Me! The Movie,* and every year we run at least one *Super Juice Me!* month, dedicated to those wishing to Super Juice themselves. I am hoping to open a *Super Juice Me Juice Camp* somewhere in the world, dedicated to people who need this approach. Watch this space!

2. KEEP ON MOVING!

By living on nothing but freshly extracted juices for 28 days, the chances are you will see some very good results. However, add exercise into the mix and those results go from very good to mind blowing. This doesn't just help to accelerate weight loss and tone the body, but for health conditions, exercise, in my opinion, is just as important as the juice, if not more important.

The number of studies that have been conducted on exercise and how it benefits every aspect of mental and physical health could fill a tome of its own, but we don't have room for this here. The most recent study (at the time of writing) estimates that one-in-six deaths are due to a lack of exercise and that inactivity is as harmful as smoking. Public Health England, the agency responsible for tackling obesity, warns that our sedentary lifestyles are not only causing obesity, they are also directly responsible for muscle and joint complaints, depression, high blood pressure, heart disease, dementia, stroke and type 2 diabetes. Professor Kevin Fenton says, 'Physical inactivity is a leading contributor to rising levels of many long term conditions. If physical activity were a drug we'd be hailing it as a miracle cure.'

Please do not underestimate the health and fitness powers of regular exercise. I not only think it's more than a good idea on the plan, but a must.

There are 10 main reasons for adding exercise into the equation on the *Super Juice Me! Challenge*. Exercise:

    i   Keeps your metabolism firing on all cylinders
    ii Helps to keep your lymph system pumping
    iii Helps to oxygenate your blood stream
    iv Helps your mood
    v   Helps you to sleep
    vi Improves your memory
    vii Helps your posture
    viii Gives you energy
    ix Helps to keep your bones strong

And, finally – and perhaps the best reason for many:

    x   You'll have better sex!

As you are only having four juices or smoothies a day, there is a chance your metabolism could slow down during the *Super Juice Me! 28-Day Juice Plan*. By adding exercise you will keep the fire burning, so to speak. This not only helps to 'condense success' during the month, but it also means that when you do go back to eating your metabolism will still be rocking.

For maximum results, make sure you exercise for around 30 minutes, *twice* a day. And when I say exercise, I don't mean you should just walk around the gym talking to your friends and checking your texts and Twitter every two minutes – I've seen you! I mean that you should work out until you sweat, really sweat.

Please do not make the very common mistake of thinking you need massive amounts of fuel before a 30-minute workout in the morning. If you are doing this to lose weight because you are packing plenty of extra pounds, then trust me, you have enough *fuel* in storage to keep you going! It's this very *fuel* you want shot of. The reason for no food before the morning workout is so you get into *fat burning* and not *sugar burning* mode.

It is also extremely important, if you only have one hour available a day for exercise, not to do the full hour at once but to break it into two, if you can. Research has shown that doing two separate high-intensity workouts a day will have a longer after-burn effect and will be around *40 per cent more effective* in terms of weight loss than if you did the full hour just in the morning or just in the evening.

If you think you can't fit it in, remember: DITCH THE EXCUSES! It's funny how the same people who tell you they don't have the time to exercise, can tell you what's going on in at least one TV soap opera or what has happened in a big box set, like 24 – which takes up...well, 24 hours of your life! (And for any pedantic 24 fans, please don't write in explaining that each episode of 24 is less than an hour because they allow for adverts. Just go with the analogy!)

3. GET THE RIGHT JUICER!

Nothing will put a nail in your juicing coffin faster than getting the wrong juicer. There are some very good juicers on the market now and some very bad ones. If you have an old juicer knocking about in a cupboard, one which doesn't allow you to feed whole apples in for example, it's time to get into 21st century juicing and upgrade. You'll be pleased you did. This is one area you shouldn't compromise on. The wrong juicer can put you off juicing for life, so please heed this piece of advice.

There are three main types of juicers:

A Fast (centrifugal)
B Slow (masticating)
C Fusion (low induction)

If you have more time on your hands, you may want to get a masticating juicer, or 'slow juicer' as they are otherwise known. (And always be careful how you say 'masticating'.) This type of juicer creates less heat friction, which usually makes for a better quality juice. The challenge is that they are often hard to clean, quite expensive and, as the name suggests, slow to use. Having said that this area is improving and the **Retro Slow Juicer** has taken this type of juicing to another level by allowing you to fit a whole apple in (something you could never do before with a slow juicer).

At the time of writing this book there is a rather large

scientific argument brewing between slow and fast juicing. There are those who claim the fruit or veg comes into contact with the fast spinning blade on a high-powered centrifugal juicer for such a short period of time that the quality of the juice isn't compromised. However, as an experiment after reading this, I made some apple-and-carrot juice in a fast juicer and some in a slow juicer. The juice made in the fast juicer immediately started to separate and become almost see-through at the bottom. The juice made in the slower juicer remained intact, even two days later! The separation is caused by oxidation, and oxidation can be caused by heat friction. Slow juicers have less heat friction and so the juice appears to be of better quality. The challenge, though, is that they are more expensive than fast juicers and usually not easy to clean.

Fast juicers, or 'centrifugal juicers' as they are otherwise known, are the most common type of juicer by far. This is because they are, as the name suggests, fast! They whizz round at anything up to 15,000 rpm (revolutions per minute), whereas a slow juicer like the **Retro** can turn at just 65 rpm. The 15,000 rpm can rip through produce in milliseconds. Many fast juicers are now pretty easy to clean too, and they are often much cheaper than the slow juicers. All these reasons add up to why they are the most popular type of juicer. There are disadvantages though. This type of juicer tends to be loud, the 'pulp' tends to be wetter, and the quality of juice lower than with a slow juicer.

But now you have the relatively new kid on the block: fusion or low-induction juicing. I say relatively new because it's new in terms of finally getting some traction within the wider juicing market. The late great juicing pioneer and 'Godfather of Fitness' Jack LaLanne brought out a juicer years ago that was 'low induction' and produced a wonderful juice. Then whole-fruit fast juicers came on the market and it appeared it was the end for low-induction juicing, until the **Fusion Juicer** range appeared. As people get more and more aware that not all juicers are built the same, quality of juice is becoming more and more important and is one of the many reasons fusion juicing is taking off. As the name suggests, it's a *fusion* of fast and slow juicing, and I believe it will end up being the most used form of juicing in years to come. Like a fast juicer, a Fusion Juicer can take whole fruit without chopping, but at just 3,000 rpm it doesn't create anywhere near as much heat friction. Remember, a fast juicer turns at about 15,000 rpm and a slow juicer at as low as 110 rpm. The Fusion Juicer sits closer to the slower end, but yet is easy to clean like most fast juicers, fits whole apples and turns out a very good quality juice. The Fusion Juicer is also extremely cheap for what it is. This is the juicer I use on the *Super Juice Me!* app and DVD. By the time you read this a newer version of the Fusion Juicer will no doubt already be on the market.

Please beware though, it's a different type of juicer, so if you are used to super-fast juicing, it may take you a short while to get your head around this halfway house. Once you have, though, you'll be pleased you did.

You will notice that all the morning and evening recipes require a blender as well as your juicer. The reason why I don't focus anywhere near as much on making suggestions about the right blender is because, unlike juicers, most blenders tend to be good. Not only that, but the chances are you already own a good blender. It's a kitchen device that most of us have – unlike a juicer. I personally use the **Fusion Booster**, not only because I like things to match in my kitchen, but also because it doubles up as a drinking bottle, so I can just blend and go! But any blender will do the trick.

The product making waves at the time of writing is the **Nutribullet**. On the original advert it said (you have to do an American infomercial voice-over here), 'It's not a juicer. It's not a blender…'. This was a strange start as it is a blender. It's like the Fusion Booster or the **Retro Blend'n'Go**, but way more expensive. I have no doubt it's a good product, but it's not a juicer and you need a juicer *and* blender/booster for this plan.

By the time you read this though, things in the juicer and blender market may well have changed again. If you think about it, the chances are you won't have the same smart phone as you had two years ago. That's because technology is constantly evolving, and it's exactly the same in the juicer business. You never know, the self-cleaning juicer (the holy grail of future juicing, we all hope) may well be with us. My advice BEFORE YOU BUY A JUICER is to jump to the www.juicemaster.com or www.superjuiceme.com websites to see what's best in the market right now.

4. FEELING HUNGRY? SOS TO THE RESCUE!

At some point during the *Super Juice Me! 28-Day Juice Plan* you may well have a couple of '**I NEED FOOD!**' moments. During the first week in particular these 'hunger moments' can arise quite a bit during the main withdrawal period from refined sugars, fats, caffeine and the like. It's worth knowing that these are in fact 'withdrawal hungers' or 'false hungers', and not genuine hunger. Withdrawal hungers manifest themselves as empty, insecure feelings, which are often identical to a normal, genuine hunger – which is why they can confuse people. This is why I advocate not using your 'Hunger SOS' until after the first five days. That way all withdrawal hungers will have subsided and you'll be in a position to know if it's a genuine hunger. Please know that you will not be lacking during the first five days if you don't use your Hunger SOS. The juices and thick blends contain everything you will need. However, if you get to the point where it's a case of either using your Hunger SOS card during the first few days or throwing in the towel, then grab your SOS!

Also bear in mind that I'm writing this for everyone. If you are a 6ft 5in athlete who trains three times a day, use your common sense and take on board an extra juice or use your SOS. The vast majority of people, even if you work out twice a day, should be OK with just the juices provided.

As the name suggests it's an 'emergency' SOS. With this in mind, once a day after 5.00pm (ideally) you can eat an emergency avocado, banana, a small handful of berries or a good natural food bar, like *Juice In A Bar* or the *Simply Nude* range of raw energy bars. Personally, I would always choose either an avocado or a veggie *Juice In A Bar*. A nice ripe avocado with lemon juice and some cracked black pepper really hits the spot; it's the most nutritious fruit on the planet and the good fats help to curb any hunger within 5 to 15 minutes.

The thing that hits the mark beautifully, especially during

the evenings, is a veggie *Juice In A Bar* and a large mug of peppermint tea with a small teaspoon of Manuka honey. In fact, for many, this Hunger SOS is their saving grace. I really look forward to this in the evenings, and every time I do any juice plan I have a veggie bar and peppermint tea on the odd evening. It more than takes the edge off; it really satisfies. I spent over a year developing what I believe to the most nutritious and natural energy bar on the market today. It also won *Best New Food Product of the Year* award at the Natural & Organic Trade Show in London.

Clearly there are many other perfectly good raw energy bars on the market, so please shop around, and have any that float your boat with your evening herbal tea. I am biased clearly, but choose your Hunger SOS wisely, and make sure it's 100 per cent raw, with no added nasties. In other words, don't choose a donut! You are more than welcome to also choose a handful of natural nuts instead of an avocado, banana or health bar.

Important note to all the cheeky ones out there: the SOS card is not transferable to other days! So, if by Friday you haven't had an SOS, don't think you can eat 5 avocados or 5 *Juice In A Bars* that day. Ideally you won't ever use your SOS card; it is there for emergency situations. This is *Super Juice Me!*, not Super 'Juice In A Bar' Me!

5. JUICE THE MIND AS WELL AS THE BODY!

I have repeatedly said this throughout this book, and it's a theme throughout all of my books. I honestly believe you cannot get into the right frame of body without first getting into the right frame of mind. Nothing will get you into the right frame of mind to start better than watching the film the plan is based on, *Super Juice Me!* And nothing will help to make sure you complete the plan better than the coaching on the 28-Day Plan app or DVD. I would challenge anyone to watch this film and not be totally inspired to 'Super Juice' themselves in some way. In fact, the chances are the film is the very reason why you find yourself reading this book right now.

Whether you have already seen the film or not, please make a point of watching it (either for the first time or again) the night before you start this plan. You want to make this as easy as possible for yourself and watching the film just before you start will make the first week easier and keep you inspired – it's all about the right frame of mind.

What you don't want is to buy all the fruit and vegetables, juicer, blender, etc., and then find you're munching on fish'n'chips on day 8! In order for you to complete this *28-Day juice plan* you need every tool at your disposal to keep you focused and in the right frame of mind. This is why I also strongly advise you to get the 28-Day Plan app or DVD. As already mentioned, I have done weekly coaching and also SOS videos to keep you on track; it's like having a 'coach in your pocket'. It's not essential, clearly, and you have the full plan here in this book, along with all the Q & As and everything you need – but never underestimate just how much the mind will need feeding as well as the body. In fact without getting the mind right, the body cannot follow.

I would also *highly* recommend feeding the mind with health documentaries such as *Food Matters*, *Hungry for Change* and the like. On that note, the makers of the two aforementioned documentaries have set up a type of 'Netflix' for health films. There's a link from www.superjuiceme.com and you can stream all films of this genre in one place. There are now many health documentaries, and the more of this information you can flood into your mind during this *28-Day juice plan* the better.

6. REST YOUR MIND & BODY!

When I was covered from head-to-toe in the skin condition psoriasis, I noticed that after a good night's sleep my skin would be far less red, flaky and fiery. Conversely, after a night on the drink and junk food and a restless night of broken sleep my skin would flare up like crazy.

When you fall into a beautiful deep sleep you are effectively recharging yourself; it's like plugging yourself in overnight in order to power up for the next day. While you sleep, the body also has time to rejuvenate and repair. A good sleep or rest is just as important as good nutrition and physical exercise, if not more so. Unfortunately, good sleep, just like good nutrition and exercise, is an area many often struggle with. Often the reason so many of us fail to get a really good night's sleep is due to either the *false stimulants* we consume daily (such as caffeine, refined sugars, fats and food chemicals), watching TV, being on the internet till late, or not doing enough in the day – such as physical exercise. Because of one of these factors or a combination of them all very rarely, if ever, does your body get a full, good night's sleep.

The good news is that I get more emails from people saying their insomnia has vanished or improved because of a juice-only programme, than about almost anything else. This is because they have no stimulants going into their bloodstream keeping them awake throughout the night. It is also because they are doing the two daily sessions of exercise I advise.

You may find that during the first three days you are disproportionately tired at times. It is not uncommon for people go to bed extremely early on the evening of night 2 and sleep non-stop for 10-12 hours. Please note this is simply down to the *withdrawal* from the false stimulants, such as refined sugars, refined fats, caffeine and the like. This will usually be gone in 72 hours, after which most people start to experience what is known as a 'juice high'. With no stimulants coming in, the body taps into its own natural energy reserves, meaning your energy is no longer of the nervous variety, but natural instead. It is also usually from day 4 or 5 onwards that you start finding yourself getting some very good nights' sleep. It is a good idea to get into the habit of turning off all screens (TVs, iPads, computers) and putting on some type of sleep-inducing music at bedtime. There are many extremely good sleep apps out there – and they can be spookily good. Paul McKenna and Glenn Harold have perhaps the best. Paul found out early on in his career that, when he started to speak, people fell asleep! So he's now put that talent to good use with his sleep apps and with seemingly old-school CDs. (BTW, that was a joke, Paul)

7. AVOID OVER THE COUNTER DRUGS!

If you are on any prescribed medication, always consult your doctor before embarking on any plan of this nature and, obviously, do not come off any prescribed drugs unless your doctor advises you to. However, if you are an OCD pill popper, my advice would be to *detox* from those too while you are on the plan (and beyond, ideally). What I mean by an OCD *pill popper* is 'over-the-counter drugs'. If you were to pick up the average person walking down the street in the UK and shake them, they would rattle. We almost have OCD about OCDs: that's Obsessive Compulsive Disorder about over-the-counter drugs. We are popping drugs without questioning what we are doing. As already mentioned, we have reached the stage where unconsciously we think a headache is caused by a lack of aspirin. The irony is that more and more research is coming forward which shows how headache tablets can actually be the cause of some people's constant headaches.

We spend almost £600 million ($840 billion) on over-the-counter drugs a year in the UK alone, this adds up to almost ONE BILLION purchases. The global market for over-the-counter drugs is expected to surpass £50 billion ($70 billion) by 2015. According to estimates from the Consumer Healthcare Products Association, retail sales of over-the-counter medicines in the US in 2010 were worth $17 billion. In my opinion, the vast majority of these drugs are being taken totally unnecessarily. Once again though, and I want to make this very clear, if you are taking any drugs, including OCDs, as part of doctor's orders, then speak to your doctor first, before stopping them.

8. EVERYONE WANTS A HOTTIE!

The vast majority of people in the UK believe they can't make it through the day without their daily cup of tea or coffee. These are 100 per cent no-no's on the plan. However, I recognize we sometimes need something hot, so here's my suggestion.

Peppermint tea (or the like) should become your new best friend over the next 28 days. If you usually go into Starbucks (other coffee chains are available), still go, but instead of your usual milkshake and sugar with a little added coffee (which, let's face it, is what the vast majority of people order), have a peppermint tea. The trick is to go for the large size (or Vente, as they call it – the word *large* would be far too simple!), ask for two teabags, leave them in and ask for a few ice cubes (they serve it while it's still boiling!). You can even have a little honey for sweetness, if you must. Who knows, by the end of the plan you may not even bother to go back to coffee or normal tea. Peppermint tea:

A   actually tastes good;

B   is light and refreshing and 100 per cent calorie free;

C   is so much cheaper than a latte!

So if you fancy a little hottie to help you through the *Super Juice Me! 28-Day Challenge*, try herbal or fruit teas.

Green tea, although it contains caffeine, is good to go on the plan. Caffeine in green tea works differently in the body because, unlike coffee, green tea also contains L-theanine. Theanine is an amino acid that produces a calming effect on the brain (Yokogoshi et al. 1998b). Japanese researchers have discovered that theanine is a caffeine antagonist, offsetting the 'hyper' effect of caffeine (Kakuda et al. 2000). Of the 20 different types of amino acids in tea, more than 60 per cent are theanine. This is unique to green tea and white tea, because the steaming process does not eliminate it. Theanine also provides the elegant taste and sweetness in green tea. It is loaded with antioxidants and actually aids weight loss, so if that's one of your goals, green tea may be the order of the day.

9. GO ORGANIC WHERE POSSIBLE!

I have made a point of saying 'where possible'. I fully understand it isn't always possible to go organic. There is a large cost often associated with it. However, it's not always cost alone which can prevent someone from going organic. Organic produce isn't always available all year round, and it depends on which country you are in, too.

I have mentioned organic produce because many of you will be doing this particular plan because of ill health, obesity, or a combination of the two. I have mentioned time and time again that the cause, in my opinion, of most lifestyle diseases comes down to two things: toxicity and deficiency. Some non-organic produce has been sprayed with all kinds of chemicals and, because the soil it was grown in is often void of certain nutrients, it can be lower on nutritional value too. Having said that please do not think for one second that an apple that has been sprayed is worse than a soda, burger and fries! You can easily Super Juice yourself non-organically, and you'll still have amazing results. I am just saying that, if you can afford it and it is available to you, why not get organic produce? This is a pure health plan you are on, so don't compromise if you don't have to. If you can't do the organic thing, simply soak your veggies in white wine vinegar before eating them. It helps to lift off any unwanted residue from sprays.

What I will also add is that most supermarkets now do organic apples and carrots and these days only slightly more expensive than non-organic. As many of the juice bases contain apple, it's worth at least using organic apples, even if you cannot get hold of anything else organic.

So to reiterate, there are two main reasons for going organic:

A Studies have shown that organic produce contains on average 40 per cent more nutrition than non-organic produce.
B You won't be ingesting the often harmful pesticides, herbicides and fungicides.

If you really can't get hold of or afford organic produce, do not despair. There are many good local farms which, although not always certified as organic producers, use much fewer chemicals than mass-market supermarket chains. Although I try to use organic produce where possible, I am also aware that even non-organic fruits and vegetables still contain a great deal more nutrients than a donut! If I'm not using organic I always Super Juice It at the same time (see tip 10).

10. SUPER JUICE IT!

If you are not going to use a great deal of organic produce, I would recommend adding some supplements in the form of Power Greens to your morning and evening juices. These are the *thicker* juices and the super green powders can be blended in. Power Greens are a powder of dried super-foods, such as whole-leaf barley grass, whole-leaf wheatgrass, nettle leaf, alfalfa leaf juice, dandelion leaf juice, barley grass juice, oat grass juice, burdock root, broccoli juice, kale juice, spinach juice, parsley juice, ginger root, spirulina, chlorella, or kelp, as well as digestive enzymes and friendly bacteria.

They are a perfect addition to this plan when you aren't sure of the nutritional value of some of the fruits and vegetables you are using. If you are getting everything organic there is no need to use these types of powders, but if you want to raise the game nutritionally, add some super greens. Power Green powders are not like vitamin and mineral tablets; they are dried foods. You might not see this powder as food, but your body very much will. There are many brands on the market, but Juice Master's Power Greens (previously Juice Master's Ultimate Superfood) are very good. I already hear you shouting, 'Yes, but you would say that wouldn't you, as that's your brand!' There are many other green powders on the market, some very good, so feel free to get any one you wish. Just do your research and make sure you are getting the real deal, otherwise it's not worth your time or money. I searched for two years to find the right combination of super-green powders and I know just how good ours are, so I make no apologies for recommending them.

You may find you love the juices without the powder and hate them with. If this is the case, leave the powder out and have it separately in water. Just add to a bottle of water, shake it and drink. It's an acquired taste, but as all the juices are so delicious it's a nice reminder that you are on a detox.

Sometimes if it's too easy and everything tastes too wonderful, we aren't convinced it's doing us any good!

A FAT LOT OF GOOD: I would also recommend, especially if you have a skin issue, adding some extra essential fatty acids to your thickies. There are several brands but Udo's cold-pressed oil blend is particularly good (no I don't get paid to endorse it!). Omega-3 & 6 essential fats are just that, *essential* for health, and your body cannot synthesize them from the foods we eat. We must directly consume these oils. Most people simply don't consume enough omega oils, so adding a spoon to your daily thickies is a simple way to address this potential deficiency.

GOOD BACTERIA are my final suggestion to have every morning on this plan. Unlike the Power Greens and oil, which are optional, I'd like to move the good bacteria to the 'must be part of the plan' category. Gut health is *everything*, and you need the right balance of 'good' and 'bad' bacteria in your gut in order to have optimum health. Good bacteria can be found in any good health food store these days. In all likelihood you will only do the *Super Juice Me! Challenge* once in your life, so I firmly believe that if you are going to do it, you should DO IT RIGHT! If you can afford it, add greens, oil and bacteria everyday to make sure you are maximizing the opportunity. It's your call on the Power Greens and the oil, if you can have everything. But if you can only have one, get those bacteria in!

THE
28-DAY
JUICE
PLAN

10

NOTE: If you wish to see the full plan at a glance with all the recipes and how to make, I recommend getting hold of the *Super Juice Me!* wall-planner. All the information is here clearly, but for those who wish to make life a great deal easier for themselves, the wall-planner comes in very useful. You can find it at **www.superjuiceme.com**

DAY 1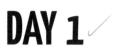

First thing: Hot water with lemon

THE GINGER SHOT (page 196)

2 x Friendly Bacteria Capsules

9am   **Juice 1:** PROTEIN RICH POWERHOUSE (page 212)

1pm   **Juice 2:** BREATH OF FRESH AIR! (page 220)

4pm   **Juice 3:** BREATH OF FRESH AIR!

7pm   **Juice 4:** PROTEIN RICH POWERHOUSE

★   ★   ★

DAY 2

First thing: Hot water with lemon

NATURAL ELECTROLYTE SODIUM SHOT (page 197)

2 x Friendly Bacteria Capsules

9am   **Juice 1:** PURE RAW ENERGY SMOOTHIE (page 210)

1pm   **Juice 2:** CHLOROPHYLL CLEANSER (page 228)

4pm   **Juice 3:** CHLOROPHYLL CLEANSER

7pm   **Juice 4:** PURE RAW ENERGY SMOOTHIE

DAY 3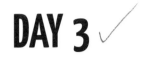

First thing: Hot water with lemon
THE GINGER SHOT (page 196)
2 x Friendly Bacteria Capsules
9am   **Juice 1:** SWEET 'N' SMOOTH VEGGIE BLEND
(page 208)
1pm   **Juice 2:** DIGESTIVE AID (page 230)
4pm   **Juice 3:** DIGESTIVE AID
7pm   **Juice 4:** SWEET 'N' SMOOTH VEGGIE BLEND

★   ★   ★

DAY 4

First thing: Hot water with lemon
NATURAL ELECTROLYTE SODIUM SHOT (page 197)
2 x Friendly Bacteria Capsules
9am   **Juice 1:** ANTIOXIDANT KING (page 204)
1pm   **Juice 2:** MINERAL MEDICINE (page 218)
4pm   **Juice 3:** MINERAL MEDICINE
7pm   **Juice 4:** ANTIOXIDANT KING

DAY 5

First thing: Hot water with lemon
THE GINGER SHOT (page 196)
2 x Friendly Bacteria Capsules

9am   **Juice 1:** ANTI-INFLAMMATORY GREEN BLEND
(page 202)
1pm   **Juice 2:** RAINBOW REMEDY (page 226)
4pm   **Juice 3:** RAINBOW REMEDY
7pm   **Juice 4:** ANTI-INFLAMMATORY GREEN BLEND

* SOAK THE ALMONDS FOR THE WEEKEND'S 'SPECIAL
GUEST' RECIPES

★   ★   ★

DAY 6

First thing: Hot water with lemon
NATURAL ELECTROLYTE SODIUM SHOT (page 197)
2 x Friendly Bacteria Capsules

9am   **Juice 1:** FIBRE OPTICS (page 200)
1pm   **Juice 2:** THE DIURETIC ONE (page 222)
4pm   **Juice 3:** THE DIURETIC ONE
7pm   **Juice 4:** TAHINI COCOA BEANEY (page 238)

DAY 7

First thing: Hot water with lemon

THE GINGER SHOT (page 196)

2 x Friendly Bacteria Capsules

9am   **Juice 1:** GREEN ZESTY SUPER SMOOTHIE (page 206)

1pm   **Juice 2:** ENERGY EXPLOSION (page 232)

4pm   **Juice 3:** ENERGY EXPLOSION

7pm   **Juice 4:** FOR GOODNESS SHAKE (page 240)

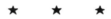

DAY 8

First thing: Hot water with lemon

NATURAL ELECTROLYTE SODIUM SHOT (page 197)

2 x Friendly Bacteria Capsules

9am   **Juice 1:** OXYGEN ELIXIR (page 214)

1pm   **Juice 2:** MINERAL MEDICINE (page 218)

4pm   **Juice 3:** MINERAL MEDICINE

7pm   **Juice 4:** OXYGEN ELIXIR

DAY 9

First thing: Hot water with lemon

THE GINGER SHOT (page 196)

2 x Friendly Bacteria Capsules

9am   **Juice 1:** PROTEIN RICH POWERHOUSE (page 212)

1pm   **Juice 2:** DIGESTIVE AID (page 230)

4pm   **Juice 3:** DIGESTIVE AID

7pm   **Juice 4:** PROTEIN RICH POWERHOUSE

★   ★   ★

DAY 10

First thing: Hot water with lemon

NATURAL ELECTROLYTE SODIUM SHOT (page 197)

2 x Friendly Bacteria Capsules

9am   **Juice 1:** FIBRE OPTICS (page 200)

1pm   **Juice 2:** CHLOROPHYLL CLEANSER (page 228)

4pm   **Juice 3:** CHLOROPHYLL CLEANSER

7pm   **Juice 4:** FIBRE OPTICS

DAY 11

First thing: Hot water with lemon

THE GINGER SHOT (page 196)

2 x Friendly Bacteria Capsules

9am   **Juice 1:** ANTIOXIDANT KING (page 204)

1pm   **Juice 2:** THE DIURETIC ONE (page 222)

4pm   **Juice 3:** THE DIURETIC ONE

7pm   **Juice 4:** ANTIOXIDANT KING

★   ★   ★

DAY 12

First thing: Hot water with lemon

NATURAL ELECTROLYTE SODIUM SHOT (page 197

2 x Friendly Bacteria Capsules

9am   **Juice 1:** PURE RAW ENERGY SMOOTHIE (page 210)

1pm   **Juice 2:** CALCIUM REFRESHER (page 224)

4pm   **Juice 3:** CALCIUM REFRESHER

7pm   **Juice 4:** PURE RAW ENERGY SMOOTHIE

* SOAK THE ALMONDS FOR THE WEEKEND'S 'SPECIAL
GUEST' RECIPES

DAY 13

First thing: Hot water with lemon

THE GINGER SHOT (page 196)

2 x Friendly Bacteria Capsules

9am   **Juice 1:** SWEET 'N' SMOOTH VEGGIE BLEND
        (page 208)

1pm   **Juice 2:** BREATH OF FRESH AIR! (page 220)

4pm   **Juice 3:** BREATH OF FRESH AIR!

7pm   **Juice 4:** SPIRULINA PROTEIN POWER SHAKE
        (page 242)

★   ★   ★

DAY 14

First thing: Hot water with lemon

NATURAL ELECTROLYTE SODIUM SHOT (page 197

2 x Friendly Bacteria Capsules

9am   **Juice 1:** OXYGEN ELIXIR (page 214)

1pm   **Juice 2:** ENERGY EXPLOSION (page 232)

4pm   **Juice 3:** ENERGY EXPLOSION

7pm   **Juice 4:** SWEET VANILLA SHAKE (page 244)

DAY 15

First thing: Hot water with lemon

THE GINGER SHOT (page 196)

2 x Friendly Bacteria Capsules

9am   **Juice 1:** PROTEIN RICH POWERHOUSE (page 212)

1pm   **Juice 2:** BREATH OF FRESH AIR! (page 220)

4pm   **Juice 3:** BREATH OF FRESH AIR!

7pm   **Juice 4:** PROTEIN RICH POWERHOUSE

★   ★   ★

DAY 16

First thing: Hot water with lemon

NATURAL ELECTROLYTE SODIUM SHOT (page 197

2 x Friendly Bacteria Capsules

9am   **Juice 1:** PURE RAW ENERGY SMOOTHIE (page 210)

1pm   **Juice 2:** CHLOROPHYLL CLEANSER (page 228)

4pm   **Juice 3:** CHLOROPHYLL CLEANSER

7pm   **Juice 4:** PURE RAW ENERGY SMOOTHIE

DAY 17

First thing: Hot water with lemon
             THE GINGER SHOT (page 196)
             2 x Friendly Bacteria Capsules
9am   **Juice 1:** SWEET 'N' SMOOTH VEGGIE BLEND
             (page 208)
1pm   **Juice 2:** DIGESTIVE AID (page 230)
4pm   **Juice 3:** DIGESTIVE AID
7pm   **Juice 4:** SWEET 'N' SMOOTH VEGGIE BLEND

★   ★   ★

DAY 18

First thing: Hot water with lemon
             NATURAL ELECTROLYTE SODIUM SHOT (page 197
             2 x Friendly Bacteria Capsules
9am   **Juice 1:** ANTIOXIDANT KING (page 204)
1pm   **Juice 2:** MINERAL MEDICINE (page 218)
4pm   **Juice 3:** MINERAL MEDICINE
7pm   **Juice 4:** ANTIOXIDANT KING

DAY 19

First thing: Hot water with lemon
THE GINGER SHOT (page 196)
2 x Friendly Bacteria Capsules

9am   **Juice 1:** ANTI-INFLAMMATORY GREEN BLEND
(page 202)

1pm   **Juice 2:** RAINBOW REMEDY (page 226)

4pm   **Juice 3:** RAINBOW REMEDY

7pm   **Juice 4:** ANTI-INFLAMMATORY GREEN BLEND

* SOAK THE ALMONDS FOR THE WEEKEND'S 'SPECIAL
GUEST' RECIPES

★   ★   ★

DAY 20

First thing: Hot water with lemon
NATURAL ELECTROLYTE SODIUM SHOT (page 197)
2 x Friendly Bacteria Capsules

9am   **Juice 1:** FIBRE OPTICS (page 200)

1pm   **Juice 2:** THE DIURETIC ONE (page 222)

4pm   **Juice 3:** THE DIURETIC ONE

7pm   **Juice 4:** TAHINI COCOA BEANEY

DAY 21

First thing: Hot water with lemon

THE GINGER SHOT (page 196)

2 x Friendly Bacteria Capsules

9am   **Juice 1:** GREEN ZESTY SUPER SMOOTHIE (page 206)

1pm   **Juice 2:** ENERGY EXPLOSION (page 232)

4pm   **Juice 3:** ENERGY EXPLOSION

7pm   **Juice 4:** FOR GOODNESS SHAKE (page 240)

★   ★   ★

DAY 22

First thing: Hot water with lemon

NATURAL ELECTROLYTE SODIUM SHOT (page 197)

2 x Friendly Bacteria Capsules

9am   **Juice 1:** OXYGEN ELIXIR (page 214)

1pm   **Juice 2:** MINERAL MEDICINE (page 218)

4pm   **Juice 3:** MINERAL MEDICINE

7pm   **Juice 4:** OXYGEN ELIXIR

DAY 23

First thing: Hot water with lemon
              THE GINGER SHOT (page 196)
              2 x Friendly Bacteria Capsules
9am   **Juice 1:** PROTEIN RICH POWERHOUSE (page 212)
1pm   **Juice 2:** DIGESTIVE AID (page 230)
4pm   **Juice 3:** DIGESTIVE AID
7pm   **Juice 4:** PROTEIN RICH POWERHOUSE

★   ★   ★

DAY 24

First thing: Hot water with lemon
              NATURAL ELECTROLYTE SODIUM SHOT (page 197)
              2 x Friendly Bacteria Capsules
9am   **Juice 1:** FIBRE OPTICS (page 200)
1pm   **Juice 2:** CHLOROPHYLL CLEANSER (page 228)
4pm   **Juice 3:** CHLOROPHYLL CLEANSER
7pm   **Juice 4:** FIBRE OPTICS

DAY 25

First thing: Hot water with lemon

THE GINGER SHOT (page 196)

2 x Friendly Bacteria Capsules

9am   **Juice 1:** ANTIOXIDANT KING (page 204)

1pm   **Juice 2:** THE DIURETIC ONE (page 222)

4pm   **Juice 3:** THE DIURETIC ONE

7pm   **Juice 4:** ANTIOXIDANT KING

★   ★   ★

DAY 26

First thing: Hot water with lemon

NATURAL ELECTROLYTE SODIUM SHOT (page 197)

2 x Friendly Bacteria Capsules

9am   **Juice 1:** PURE RAW ENERGY SMOOTHIE (page 210)

1pm   **Juice 2:** CALCIUM REFRESHER (page 224)

4pm   **Juice 3:** CALCIUM REFRESHER

7pm   **Juice 4:** PURE RAW ENERGY SMOOTHIE

* SOAK THE ALMONDS FOR THE WEEKEND'S 'SPECIAL
GUEST' RECIPES

DAY 27

First thing: Hot water with lemon
            THE GINGER SHOT (page 196)
            2 x Friendly Bacteria Capsules
9am   **Juice 1:** SWEET 'N' SMOOTH VEGGIE BLEND
                (page 208)
1pm   **Juice 2:** BREATH OF FRESH AIR! (page 220)
4pm   **Juice 3:** BREATH OF FRESH AIR!
7pm   **Juice 4:** SPIRULINA PROTEIN POWER SHAKE
                (page 242)

★   ★   ★

DAY 28

First thing: Hot water with lemon
            NATURAL ELECTROLYTE SODIUM SHOT (page 197
            2 x Friendly Bacteria Capsules
9am   **Juice 1:** OXYGEN ELIXIR (page 214)
1pm   **Juice 2:** ENERGY EXPLOSION (page 232)
4pm   **Juice 3:** ENERGY EXPLOSION
7pm   **Juice 4:** SWEET VANILLA SHAKE (page 244)

LET'S GO SHOPPING!

11

BEFORE YOU NIP TO THE SHOPS READ THIS!

The Super Juice Me! 28-Day Juice Plan is effectively a 14-Day plan repeated. This is why you will notice that the shopping list for weeks 1 and 3 are identical, as to are weeks 2 and 4. Although the shopping lists in the book are week by week, you can of course choose to shop by the day or every three days, or whatever floats your shopping boat. Clearly this involves working out exactly what you will need for just 1 or 3 days etc from the recipes and this can take some time as well as good mathematics! If you have the Super Juice Me! app for Iphone and Android there is a feature which enables you to shop by the day and it works it all out for you, but for the purposes of the book you'll see just three different shopping lists:

1. Week 1 & 3
2. Week 2 & 4
3. Full 28-Days

In 'Week 1 & 3' and 'week 2 & 4' shopping lists you'll find the fresh fruit and veggies you will need for those particular weeks. The 'Full 28-Day' shopping list has the extras you will need for the whole plan. You only need to buy them once at the start as they will keep for the full 28-days, these are items such as Hemp protein powder, frozen berries, almonds, Power greens and so on. If you miss getting any of these you'll not be a camper – especially when going to make the very, very delicious Tahini Cocoa Beany, so…

MAKE SURE YOU GET THE 28-DAY SHOPPING BEFORE YOU START

You can also download the full shopping list at www. superjuiceme.com

HAPPY SHOPPING!

Week 1 & 3

32 Apples

6 spears Asparagus

5 medium/large Avocados

5 Bananas

8 bulbs raw Beetroot

1 large head & stem of Broccoli

17 medium Carrots

1 small Cauliflower

20 sticks Celery

1 Courgette (Zucchini)

6 Cucumbers

1 bulb Fennel

1 large claw Ginger

1 small bag Kale (206g)

2 Lemons

9 Limes

2 handfuls Mint (Fresh)

4 leaves Basil

2 Oranges

3 Parsnips

12 Pea pods

9 Pears

3 Pineapples

1 small Red Cabbage

1 large bag Spinach (500g)

2 Tomatoes

Week 2 & 4

35 Apples

6 spears Asparagus

4 medium/large Avocados

5 Bananas

9 bulbs raw Beetroot

19 medium Carrots

20 sticks Celery

1 Courgette (Zucchini)

6 Cucumbers

1 bulb Fennel

1 claw Ginger

1 large head & stem of Broccoli

1 small bag Kale (206g)

2 Lemons

7 Limes

4 handfuls Mint (Fresh)

8 leaves Basil

2 Oranges

3 Parsnips

12 Pea pods

8 Pears

2 Pineapples

1 large bag Spinach (500g)

1 Turnip

Full 28 Days

500g Almonds (Unsalted & Raw)

1 small bag Mixed Berries (350g if frozen)

1 large bag Mixed Seeds (350g)

2 pods Vanilla (Extract)

1 small pot Honey (pref local or Manuka)

1 small pot Cocoa Powder (fair-trade & Raw)

1 jar of Tahini (sesame seed 'butter')

4 litres Mineral Water

1 large bag Ice

1 tub of Hemp Protein Powder

56 capsules Friendly Bacteria

1 small jar Spirulina

1 small jar Powergreens (optional)

SUPER JUICE ME!

THE RECIPES

PURE LIQUID GOLD

NO ADDED SUGAR

NO ARTIFICIAL COLOURS

NO ARTIFICIAL FLAVOURINGS

NO ADDED SALT

NO REFINED FATS

NO NASTIES WHATSOEVER

11

It is hard to describe pure live juice as anything other than liquid gold. It is the most efficient bio-available form of nutrition known to us and has the potential to make us richer that any block of actual gold. As I have already pointed out, true wealth isn't gauged by what's in your bank, but rather by what you put into your body. Every time you drink a freshly extracted juice you make a sizeable deposit which goes some way to securing your future wealth. By drinking *nothing* but freshly extracted juices and smoothies for 28 days, it's like having a win on the lottery. Continue with a healthy lifestyle after the 28 days – I have made several suggestions on page 309 – and you'll earn compound interest to spend when everyone else around you starts to pay the price for not topping up their account when they had the chance.

Every juice in this plan produces a glass of liquid, brimming with vibrant colour. This colour comes only from what nature provides and it's the different colour pigmentation within all fruits and vegetables that provide us with the nutrition we need. The creamy, slightly sweet, delicious taste of the juices are a result of the natural sugars contained within the fruits and vegetables. We don't need to add anything to improve them. The thick rich texture and beautiful slightly frothy head is the sign of pure 'live' juice. You can be assured that when you make any of the fresh juices for you and your family on this plan they are all:

100% NATURAL / 100% VEGAN

100% RAW / 100% 'LIVE'

In terms of amounts to expect when making the juices in the plan, all have been designed to make a juice or smoothie of approximately 450-500ml in size. This is exactly the size we served at Juicy Oasis health retreat in Portugal when doing the *Super Juice Me! Big Juice Experiment*, the film; it's the size we use for our *Juice Master Delivered* service; and it's the perfect amount of juice per serving if you're doing nothing but a juice 'cleanse'. You may find there's be some variation on this, depending on the size of the produce you use. Not all carrots and avocados are built the same for example. I have seen avocados in some parts of the world the size of footballs and carrots the size of large cucumbers. In every recipe in this *Super Juice Me!* plan, I stipulate things like 'half an avocado' and I think it's safe to say we all know what that is roughly. It doesn't mean half of an avocado the size of a house! Organic courgettes (zucchini), as another example, can be two or three times the size of the supermarket variety. However, most people will be shopping at a supermarket so it is the average produce found here that has been used in the recipes, so please feel free to adjust accordingly.

THE
SUPER
SHOTS

THE LITTLE SHOTS
WITH THE BIG IMPACT!

THE GINGER SHOT

Makes a showing on alternate days

This is also known as the 'healthy espresso', but beware, it packs one hell of a punch. If you feel you need a greater lift than usual one morning, then simply add extra ginger, guaranteed to blow away those cobwebs! I first tasted this beauty at Jo & The Juice, a really cool juice bar chain from Denmark. Kasper, one of the founders, invited me to try it when I was over there a few years ago and I have had one every morning since. This shot appears every other day, but if you love it, feel free to have it everyday on the plan and beyond!

Juicy Ingredients
3 cm (1 inch) Ginger
1 small or ½ large Apple

Juicy Instructions
Simply juice the ingredients and knock back as a shot!

The Clever Stuff

Ginger juice is like a first aid kit in liquid form! Not only is it antifungal, antiseptic and antibacterial but it is also antiviral and a fantastic antihistamine making it the perfect tonic for anyone who suffers with hay fever or other allergies. Ginger is stimulating and helps to promote detoxification by increasing circulation; it also improves the absorption of other essential nutrients in the body.

NATURAL ELECTROLYTE SODIUM SHOT

Makes a showing on alternate days

This is a powerhouse of sodium and potassium and is imperative for replacing lost salts due to exercise, so this is a wonderful pre or post workout juice. This is also a very anti-inflammatory blend so highly recommended for arthritis and other inflammatory conditions. As part of the *Super Juice Me!* Plan it is imperative, so please don't skip it!

Juicy Ingredients
¼ medium Cucumber
1 stick Celery

Juicy Instructions
Simply juice the ingredients and knock back as a shot!

The Clever Stuff

Both celery and cucumber create the perfect balance of sodium and potassium, which works as a natural electrolyte. Electrolytes help to keep the body in balance, regulating your body's fluids and helping maintain a healthy blood pH balance. They also create the electrical impulses essential to all aspects of physical activity, from basic cell function to the complex neuromuscular interactions needed for athletic performance.

THE 'THICKIES'

Or 'Smoothies' by any other name!

FIBRE OPTICS

Makes a showing on days 6, 10, 20 and 24

Aptly named by Dan, Juicy HQ's technical wizard, this cheeky juice has a few surprises in store. A playful combination of apples cucumber and carrot, combined with fragrant basil, fiery ginger, a chunk of banana for good measure and some blended pear (just because we can!) makes this a real game changer! Enjoy

Juicy Ingredients

1 medium **Carrot** (remove hard top)
2 **Apples** (Golden Delicious or Gala)
½ medium **Cucumber**
3 cm **Ginger**
4 leaves **Basil**
¼ **Banana**
1 **Pear** (¼ diced and blended and ¾ juiced)
3 cubes **Ice**

Juicy Instructions

Juice the carrot, cucumber, ginger, apples and ¾ of the pear. Take the other ¼ of the pear and cut into chunks. Add to the blender along with the *extracted juice*, basil, banana and ice and blend for a full minute.

The Clever Stuff

If you thought it was a myth that **CARROTS** are good for the eyesight, then you would be wrong. Carrots are an exceptional source of beta-carotene, which the body converts into vitamin A. This is fundamental for good vision. Without it, the eye's photoreceptors begin to deteriorate. According to the University of Maryland Medical Centre, people who eat a lot of foods rich in vitamin A (such as fresh carrots), have a lower risk of developing cataracts than people who don't.

The **PEAR** in this recipe provides both soluble and insoluble fibre. When combined with liquid, soluble fibre forms a thick gel that helps to bind toxins and provide bulk to ensure everything keeps 'moving'. Soluble fibre slows down digestion, which keeps you feeling fuller for longer, but has also been said to help in reducing cholesterol and controlling blood sugar levels. Insoluble fibre passes through your gut without being broken down. It helps to prevent digestive problems and keep your bowels healthy and happy.

BASIL is most commonly used in cooking, but this powerful little leaf completely transforms a juice into something exciting and truly unique! The word 'basil' is actually Greek and comes from the Greek word *basileus*, which means 'king'. As well as releasing a fragrant aroma and pungent flavour, basil is widely nutritious and has an abundance of health benefits. It is rich in vitamin A, also known as retinol, which is important for healthy skin and building our immunity to disease as well as being a source of iron and other minerals.

ANTI-INFLAMMATORY GREEN BLEND

Makes a showing on days 5 and 19

Inflammation is a common cause of dis-ease within the body, which is why we have included this mellow green blend to help put out some fires. This juice contains a whole spectrum of fruits and veggies well known for their ant-inflammatory properties, but also some not so well known, like the underrated cauliflower. Hidden amongst the sweetness of juicy pineapple and pear means your body gets to reap the health benefits whilst your taste buds get to enjoy!

Juicy Ingredients
¼ medium **Pineapple** (peeled)
1 **Pear** (any hard variety)
1 **Lime** (peeled)
3 cm **Ginger**
¼ medium **Cucumber**
½ stick **Celery**
1 **Cauliflower** floret (Roughly the size of a lime)
½ medium **Avocado** (ripe)
3 cubes **Ice**

Juicy Instructions
Juice the pineapple, pear, lime, ginger, cucumber, celery and cauliflower. Add the avocado flesh and ice to a blender/booster, pour in the *extracted juice* and blend until smooth.

The Clever Stuff

Eating refined carbohydrates, sugars and dairy, etc. tends to raise inflammatory markers for most people, and most disease is linked to or caused by inflammation. Cruciferous vegetables, such as cauliflower, contain a compound called sulforaphane that has been widely studied because of its anti-inflammatory action in the body. Despite appearing acidic, pineapple is also a powerful anti-inflammatory.

PINEAPPLE is rich in vitamin C and manganese, and, most importantly, an enzyme called bromelain, which has anti-inflammatory properties that are widely used to help ease arthritic and other pains caused by inflammation.

CUCUMBER juice reduces the high uric acid content that causes inflammation in degenerative diseases such as rheumatism and arthritis, making it another natural anti-inflammatory.

The humble **CAULIFLOWER**, often overshadowed by its more popular cruciferous relation broccoli, has a wealth of health to offer. In fact the cauliflower is packed with nutrients that help to keep inflammation at bay, which is why it really holds its own in this juice. It's a great source of vitamin K and omega-3 fatty acids, both of which help to reduce inflammation. Vitamin K also acts as a direct regulator of our inflammatory responses.

ANTIOXIDANT KING

Makes a showing on days 4, 11, 18 and 25

We're mixing it up in this recipe to create a 'thickie' that packs a powerful ant-oxidant punch. Fusing the sweet treats of pineapple, apple, plump berries and banana with the earthy, savoury notes of beetroot and leafy green spinach to create a fun and filling meal in a glass.

Juicy Ingredients

¼ medium **Pineapple** (peeled)
1 **Apple** (Golden Delicious or Gala)
1 large handful **Spinach**
1 small bulb Raw **Beetroot** (remove hard ends)
1 handful **Mixed Berries** (fresh or frozen)
½ **Banana**
3 cubes **Ice**

Juicy Instructions

Juice the pineapple, apple, spinach and beetroot. Add the banana, berries, *extracted juice* and ice to the blender/booster and blend everything until smooth.

The Clever Stuff

Antioxidants are important, as they are super nutrients that fight free radical damage that can otherwise harm cells. This damage can manifest in disease and signs of ageing, hence the 'antioxidant = anti-ageing' theory. Although not technically correct, as you cannot slow down the process of ageing, you can certainly prevent it speeding up by boosting your antioxidant levels! Your body cannot produce antioxidants such as beta-carotene, lutein, lycopene, selenium and vitamins A, C and E, so you have to obtain them from plant foods:

BLUEBERRIES, blackberries and other berries are renowned for their high levels of antioxidants. They have many properties, which can be helpful in reducing the signs of ageing, by helping the skin to keep its elasticity, thus preventing wrinkles. Blackberries are packed with anthocyanins, a phytochemical that both gives them their deep glossy colour and acts as an antioxidant by helping to reduce inflammation. These rich and juicy berries are also high in vitamins, particularly vitamin A, C, E and K.

BEETS contain polyphenols and betalain, important natural antioxidants. Research over the past 10 years has been increasingly documenting the importance of polyphenols in the human diet. According to the *American Journal of Clinical Nutrition*, polyphenols, a type of antioxidant, are clinically proven to prevent cardiovascular disease in humans. Beetroot also contains betacyanin, a powerful antioxidant and pigment that gives them their deep and vibrant colour Beets are one of the richest sources of glutamine, an amino acid, essential to the health and maintenance of the intestinal tract.

GREEN ZESTY SUPER SMOOTHIE

Makes a showing on days 7 and 21

Life on earth simply wouldn't exist without the colour green; it really is the life force of Mother Nature. So what better way to start your day than with this super fusion of green goodness? Fennel adds a delicate aniseed overtone making this juice truly unique.

Juicy Ingredients
2 **Pear**s (any hard variety)
½ **Lime** (rind on)
1 cm **Fennel**
½ medium **Courgette/Zucchini**
1 stick **Celery**
1 large handful **Spinach**
½ medium **Avocado** (ripe)
3 cubes **Ice**

Juicy Instructions
Juice the pears, lime, fennel, courgette/zucchini, celery and spinach. Add the avocado flesh, *extracted juice* and ice to the blender and errr… blend!

The Clever Stuff

AVOCADOS are actually a fruit, and they have one of the highest levels of protein compared with other fruits. They are also a wonderful source of essential fatty acids, and the monounsaturated fats can help reduce cholesterol and maintain a healthy heart. Avocados are considered one of the healthiest foods on the planet because they contain in excess of 25 essential nutrients, including vitamins A, B, C, E and K, copper, iron, phosphorus, magnesium, and potassium. One of the most energy dense fruits and, gram for gram, contain 60% more potassium than bananas. Potassium is essential for the proper function of all cells, tissues, and organs in the human body.

PEARS are a great source of minerals such as iron, potassium, manganese, copper and magnesium, and also those all-important B-complex vitamins such as riboflavin (B2), folic acid (B9) and pyridoxine (B6). Pears are one of the highest fibre fruits, and their high content of the soluble fibre pectin makes them very useful in helping to lower cholesterol levels.

FENNEL is an aromatic herb and an excellent source of Vitamin C, which neutralizes free radicals that could otherwise cause cellular damage resulting in pain and disease. It is also used to aid digestion and ease bloating. Fennel is a good source of potassium, which is a key mineral known to reduce high blood pressure. Lowering blood pressure can reduce the risk of strokes and heart attacks

SWEET 'N' SMOOTH VEGGIE BLEND

Makes a showing on days 3, 13, 17 and 27

Veggies really are 'where it's at' when it comes to optimum health but they are not always the most palatable on their own. This beautiful blend of natures finest greens combined with sweet notes from the apples and parsnip, the subtle zest of lime and creaminess of avocado, really does tick all of the boxes.

Juicy Ingredients

2 **Apples** (Golden Delicious)
1 handful **Spinach**
¼ medium **Courgette/Zucchini** (remove hard ends)
1 **Lime** (peeled)
½ stalk **Celery**
¼ medium **Cucumber**
3 cm **Broccoli** stem
½ medium **Parsnip** (remove hard end)
½ medium **Avocado** (ripe)
3 cubes **Ice**

Juicy Instructions

Juice the apples, spinach, courgette/zucchini, lime, celery, cucumber, broccoli stem and parsnip. Add the avocado flesh and ice to a blender, pour in the *extracted juice* and blend until smooth.

The Clever Stuff!

PARSNIPS are a wonderful source of soluble fibre, which has been found to help keep blood sugar levels regulated and reduce cholesterol.

BROCCOLI could help in relieving the current vitamin D deficiency as it has an unusually high concentration of vitamin A and vitamin K. These vitamins are vital for helping to keep our vitamin D metabolism in balance. Like all cruciferous vegetables, broccoli promotes good colon health, protecting against constipation and colon cancer.

LIMES promote a healthy intestine, as the acid scours the intestinal tract, eliminating toxins and neutralizing harmful bacteria. Limes are an excellent source of vitamin C. In the 19th century lemons and limes were given to British sailors to help prevent scurvy, a common condition caused by a vitamin C deficiency (hence British sailors being nicknamed limeys!).

CELERY comes from the same family as parsley and fennel and one thing they all have in common is potent flavour. Try and juice the green leaves, as they contain potassium that balances the high sodium content of the stalk. Celery contains a compound called 3-n-butylphthalide, which is a powerful anti-inflammatory and natural painkiller, making it very useful for rheumatic and muscular pain. Celery is a good source of Vitamin K, an essential vitamin for normal blood clotting and healthy bones.

PURE RAW ENERGY SMOOTHIE

Makes a showing on days 2, 12, 16 and 26

When most people need an energy boost they tend to look for the nearest coffee house or chemically charged energy drink. Everything we need we can get from nature, and that includes bags of energy to keep you running throughout the day. If you don't believe me then try this delightful smoothie. I've left nothing out of this baby! Its thick and creamy, sweet and satiating and LOADED with all the good stuff your body needs.

Juicy Ingredients

1 **Apple** (Golden Delicious or Gala)

¼ medium **Pineapple** (peeled)

2 sticks **Celery**

1 large **Carrot** (remove hard end)

1 medium bulb Raw **Beetroot** (remove hard ends)

¼ Lemon (rind on, wax free)

½ medium **Banana**

½ medium **Avocado** (ripe)

1 heaped teaspoon **Hemp Protein Powder***

3 cubes **Ice**

Juicy Instructions

Juice the apple, pineapple, celery, carrot, beetroot and lemon. Pour the *extracted juice* into the blender/booster; add the banana, avocado flesh, hemp protein powder, ice and blend until smooth.

The Clever Stuff!

All raw fruits and vegetables are virtually pre-digested by the plant and therefore free up valuable energy for us to use on other activities apart from digestion. On top of this, this thickie is boosted with hemp protein powder which is loaded with essential fatty acids and, in a 3:1 ratio, exactly right for the human body. These fatty acids are broken down in a process of oxidation, which produces twice as much energy as carbohydrates or proteins. **HEMP SEEDS** contain essential amino acids. Amino acids are the building blocks of protein and they also improve muscle control, mental function and the body's maintenance of cells, muscle, tissues, and organs.

Another key ingredient in this smoothie is **BANANA**, which is essentially nature's energy bar and perhaps the single greatest energy provider nature has to offer. Bananas contain fibre, potassium and B vitamins, important nutrients that help with sustaining energy. Bananas may also help ease symptoms of depression due to their high levels of tryptophan, an amino acid which gets converted into serotonin, a monoamine neurotransmitter associated with enhancing mood and sense of well being.

---

*   Available from all good health food shops or juicemaster.com but please make sure you purchase one that is 100% hemp and no other fillers

PROTEIN RICH POWERHOUSE
Makes a showing on days 1, 9, 15 and 23

This is your first 'meal' on the *Super Juice Me!* 28-Day Plan and what a way to get you started! I haven't messed about here, straight in with plenty of mineral rich veggies, sweetened with fruit plus 'God's Butter', the avocado. But I didn't finish there; I'm raising the protein stakes by adding a cheeky bit of hemp protein powder and mixed seeds for a satisfying crunch!

Juicy Ingredients
1 **Apple** (Golden Delicious or Gala)
1 large handful **Spinach**
¼ medium **Pineapple** (peeled)
¼ medium **Cucumber**
1 **Lime** (peeled)
3 cm **Broccoli** stem
6 pods **Fresh Peas** (not cooked/frozen)
½ medium **Avocado** (ripe)
1 heaped teaspoon **Hemp Protein Powder***
1 tablespoon **Mixed Seeds*** (i.e. sunflower, pumpkin, chia)
3 cubes **Ice**

Juicy Instructions
Juice the apple, spinach, pineapple, cucumber, lime, broccoli stem and peas. Add the avocado flesh, mixed seeds, hemp protein powder and ice to the blender, pour in the *extracted juice* and blend until smooth.

The Clever Stuff!

As well as containing **HEMP**, which is one of the richest sources of readily digestible vegetable protein in the world, this thickie also contains peas, mainly because I wanted to 'give peas a chance' (I know, I know!) **PEA** protein powder is the other popular non-dairy alternative to whey protein powder. This smoothie will certainly taste better than a powdered pea or hemp protein shake and it contains a multitude of other health properties.

Mixed seeds provide an added protein boost whilst keeping your teeth occupied. According to the United States Department of Agriculture's Nutrient Database, a serving size of pumpkin seeds (which equals approximately 1/2 a cup), contains an average of 8 grams of protein. Chia, unlike many other nutritious plants, is considered to be a 'complete protein' having all 9 essential amino acids as well as other non-essential. Seeds are an excellent source of fibre and we'll carry on praising the chia seed as they contain 4-5 grams of fibre in a single teaspoon. When combined with liquid chia seeds form a thick gel that helps bind toxins, provide bulk and keep you 'moving'.

*Available from all good health food shops or juicemaster.com but please make sure you purchase one that is 100% hemp and no other fillers

**If you don't like a smoothie with 'bits' then leave out the seeds, but remember they are a great source of fibre, protein and Essential Fatty Acids.

OXYGEN ELIXIR

Makes a showing on days 8, 14, 22 and 28

It's important that the foods we eat (or drink in this case) help to bump up our body's oxygen levels. It's when our cells are deprived of oxygen that they become a breeding ground for disease. So this tasty little tonic, courtesy of Mother Nature, is just what the doctor ordered. Thick and creamy, avocado, serene celery, the slight bitter taste of lemon balanced by the sweetness of apple and carrot combined with the visual vibrancy of ruby red beetroot ...one word....divine!

Juicy Ingredients

2 **Apples** (Golden Delicious or Gala)
1 small bulb Raw **Beetroot** (remove hard ends)
1 medium **Carrot** (remove hard end)
1 stick **Celery**
¼ **Lemon** (rind on, wax free)
½ medium **Avocado** (ripe)
3 cubes **Ice**

Juicy Instructions

Juice the apples, beetroot, carrot, celery and lemon. Add the avocado flesh and ice to the blender, pour in the *extracted juice* and blend until smooth.

The Clever Stuff!

Oxygen, as we all know, is essential to sustain life. When our cells are starved of oxygen to any extent, our health begins to suffer. It is mainly absorbed through the lungs and then carried to the cells in our body via our bloodstream. We can keep our cells oxygenated through diet and the consumption of life giving, raw foods (you know, foods that haven't had been cooked to within an inch of their life!), fresh fruits and vegetables.

RAW BEETROOT juice has been found to help with oxygenation of the blood as it contains high levels of nitrates, which improve blood flow throughout the body. Nitrates help dilate blood vessels and therefore allow better oxygen absorption. Many world-class athletes are consuming beetroot juice, as it is claimed to improved exercise performance. Essentially beetroot juice allows your muscles to perform the same amount of work while using less oxygen. It can also help in rebuilding red blood cells making it an excellent source for treating iron deficiencies and anaemia. An acidic environment in the bloodstream can lead to lower oxygen levels, which is why fruit and vegetable juices are so beneficial as they are very alkalizing in the body.

LEMONS, although acidic to begin with, are actually very alkalizing and can help to restore balance to the body's pH – who knew! Lemons also have powerful antibacterial properties, which is why you will notice they are used in a lot of household cleaners.

THE 'THIN' ONES

Or Juices as they're otherwise known!

MINERAL MEDICINE

Makes a showing on days 4, 8, 18 and 22

Minerals are essential for growth and regulating bodily functions. This recipe is full of mineral rich goodness but unlike most 'medicines' it tastes delicious too. Fresh broccoli, celery and asparagus with cooling cucumber, the pungent kick of ginger and the light sweetness of parsnip and apples.

Juicy Ingredients
2 **Apples** (Golden Delicious or Gala)
3 cm **Broccoli** stem
1 stick **Celery**
¼ medium **Cucumber**
3 cm **Ginger**
1 **Asparagus** spear
1 medium **Parsnip**
3 cubes **Ice**

Juicy Instructions
Juice all the fruits and vegetables, then either pour the *extracted juice* into the blender with ice and blend or simply add ice to a glass and pour over.

The Clever Stuff!

There are two kinds of minerals: macrominerals, which include potassium, phosphorus, calcium, sodium, potassium, sulfur and magnesium, and 'trace' minerals such as manganese, zinc, manganese, iron, cobalt, fluoride, copper and selenium. Whilst elements of all are important for overall health, we need macrominerals in much higher quantities than trace minerals.

BROCCOLI is a great source of phosphorous and calcium, vital for skeletal strength. It is also abundant in the trace mineral manganese; this helps protect cells from oxidative stress, which can otherwise increases the aging process. It is also important in helping you heal after an injury.

ASPARAGUS contains a range of minerals including calcium, magnesium, phosphorus, potassium, sodium and iron. In addition, it is an anti-inflammatory and high in antioxidants, two of the best risk reducers for common chronic health problems, including type 2 diabetes and heart disease.

CELERY, well known for its cleansing properties, is also rich in sodium, an essential mineral for maintaining healthy blood pressure. Celery leaves contain iodine, a mineral that helps to promote the production of thyroid hormones that keep our cells and metabolic rate healthy.

CUCUMBERS are rich in silicon and sulphur minerals that stimulate the kidneys resulting in increased flushing out. Cucumber juice reduces the high uric acid content that causes inflammation in degenerative diseases such as rheumatism and arthritis and gout, making it a natural anti-inflammatory.

BREATH OF FRESH AIR!

Makes a showing on days 1, 13, 15 and 27

Never has a name better described a juice. The cool tones of mint offset by the warmth of spicy ginger, zesty orange and the all important 'King Carrot', all work beautifully together to create a real statement juice with such depth and vigour you'll be refreshed, energized and ready for whatever the rest of day has in store!

Juicy Ingredients
1 large **Orange** (peeled, but with the pith on)
2 medium **Carrot** (remove hard end)
1 small bulb Raw **Beetroot** (remove hard ends)
1 large handful Fresh **Mint**
3 cm **Ginger**
3 cubes **Ice**

Juicy Instructions
Juice all the fruit and vegetables, then either pour the *extracted juice* into the blender with ice and blend or simply add ice to a glass and pour over.

The Clever Stuff!

MINT is a beautiful herb that can help ease indigestion and heartburn. It can also fight the bacteria in your mouth that causes bad breath, so make sure you 'chew' this juice and drink it slowly, allowing the mint to perform its magic.

ORANGES are renowned for their vitamin C content and their consequent ability to help boost the immune system. The vitamin C also protects cells by neutralizing free radicals, which can otherwise cause chronic diseases, like cancer and heart disease.

There really is no end to the health giving benefits of **GINGER** and it will definitely be a staple in your shopping basket from here on in! It's commonly recognized as the 'king' of anti-inflammatory foods, but it also helps with nausea and feelings of motion sickness, flu symptoms, poor circulation and gastro-intestinal relief. Ginger also helps us to better absorb other essential nutrients as well. It is a great circulation stimulant due to the compounds gingerols, which cause a rapid and noticeable widening of the blood vessel walls and thus help to enhance circulation and lower blood pressure. Enhanced circulation of course means that the body can transport oxygen, nutrients and white blood cells to sites of infection more efficiently; it also enhances the removal of waste.

CARROTS are known as the anti-cancer 'kings' of the vegetable world. They contain some amazing antioxidants, including alpha-carotene, lutein, beta-carotene and lycopene, to name a few. Beta-carotene is the daddy of nutrients when it comes to its cancer preventing properties, as it is believed that beta-carotene can break down the protective mucous membrane around cancer cells.

THE DIURETIC ONE

Makes a showing on days 6, 11, 20 and 25

Does exactly what it says on the tin! There are several medical conditions that can cause your body to build up too much fluid. It's all about balance and that's where this juice comes into play. Basically, if it's not green, it's not going in! Enjoy.

Juicy Ingredients
1 medium **Pear** (any hard variety)
½ medium **Cucumber**
½ **Lime** (rind on)
2 spears **Asparagus**
1 stick **Celery**
1 large handful **Spinach**
3 cubes **Ice**

Juicy Instructions
Juice all the fruits and vegetables, then either pour the *extracted juice* into the blender with ice and blend or simply add ice to a glass and pour over.

The Clever Stuff!

High water-content fruits and vegetables, such as cucumber, celery and asparagus, help the body to flush out toxins and water through increased urination.

CUCUMBERS are rich in silicon and sulphur that stimulate the kidneys, resulting in increased flushing out. They are rich in silica, which helps strengthen connective tissues. In practical terms, this means strong hair and nails.

ASPARAGUS is 93% water and contains asparagines, which boost kidney performance and help the body remove waste and water. Asparagus is one of the richest vegetable sources of folic acid. Folic acid is a B vitamin that promotes the formation of healthy red blood cells and helps reduce the risk of neural tube defects, such as spina bifida in unborn babies. So if you know someone who's pregnant, then why not treat them to a nice bunch of asparagus? (I'm sure that will go down well!).

CELERY has been used as a natural diuretic for centuries. It contains sodium and potassium, important minerals that help to regulate the fluid balance in the body. Any excess fluid will be flushed from the body, which is helpful in reducing bloating.

LIMES may be small but they are full of flavour and will always add a certain *je-ne-sais-quoi* on the taste front. Nutritionally, one whole lime contains approximately 35 per cent of your daily vitamin C requirements. As we all know, vitamin C is key in warding off those winter colds.

PEARS are a gentler diuretic. They are a very fibrous fruit containing pectin, a gel-like substance that helps in sweeping waste and toxins from the body. Drinking pear juice can also help regulate bowel movements.

CALCIUM REFRESHER

Makes a showing on days 12 and 26

A lack of calcium can lead to all kinds of health problems including rickets and osteoporosis but that doesn't mean you need to go and suck on a cow's udder! Calcium is found in abundance in fruits and vegetables, which is excellent news considering that is what the vast majority of your 28 days is going to consist of! We've dedicated an entire juice to this mighty mineral so enjoy!

Juicy Ingredients
1 **Apple** (Golden Delicious or Gala)
1 **Pear** (any hard variety)
¼ medium **Cucumber**
1 **Lime** (peeled)
1 handful Fresh **Mint**
3 cm **Broccoli** stem
1 large handful **Spinach**
½ small **Turnip** (remove hard end)
3 cubes **Ice**

Juicy Instructions
Juice all the fruits and vegetables, then either pour the *extracted juice* into the blender with ice and blend or simply add ice to a glass and pour over.

The Clever Stuff!

As most people know, calcium is essential for the growth and strength of teeth and bones. But more than that, it is actually the main constituent in the skeleton, so it is an incredibly important mineral. When you lack calcium, the body starts to pull it from your bones and teeth, which is when problems start to occur. It is an important mineral for muscle contraction, and a deficiency can cause numbness in fingers as well as toe- and muscle-cramps.

TURNIPS? In a delicious tasting juice? YES, and rightly so, as the underused turnip has loads to offer on a nutritional level and, if used in the right quantity, on a taste level too. The bulb is rich in vitamin C, which helps to protect cells and keep them healthy. The leafy green top is fine to juice and is an excellent source of vitamins A, C and K, folic acid, and calcium.

BROCCOLI stems are so often thrown away, but are just as nutritious as the florets, which is why they should never go to waste. In fact, in juicing it's all about the stem. You'll get the same satisfaction from finding a nice thick broccoli stem as you do when you discover the nice big, perfectly ripe avocado hidden at the back of the display! Broccoli contains approximately 47mg of calcium per 100g and is easily absorbed by the body, so really helps in totting up that calcium score. It helps to strengthen our immune system and promotes healing through its powerful antioxidant properties.

SPINACH contains approximately 99mg of calcium per 100g and also boasts high levels of vitamin A, vitamin C, vitamin K, magnesium, manganese, folic acid, and iron. As if that wasn't enough, it also rich in sulforaphane, an important chemical on account of its cancer-fighting properties.

RAINBOW REMEDY

Makes a showing on days 5 and 19

This beautiful juice isn't just the pot of gold at the end of the rainbow; it is the rainbow! Every time I see the juice flooding from the juicer it never fails to amaze me the sheer depth and vibrancy of colour that exists in nature. There are certainly no added colours, dyes, preservatives or sugars in this juice, just as nature intended! It's flavours reflective of a light, fresh salad with an added twist of ginger and a squeeze of lemon. Delicious.

Juicy Ingredients

2 **Apples** (Golden Delicious or Gala)
1 medium **Carrot**
1 stick **Celery**
¼ medium **Cucumber**
1 medium bulb Raw **Beetroot**
1 small handful **Red Cabbage**
1 medium **Tomato** (remove stalk)
3 cm **Ginger**
¼ **Lemon** (rind on, wax free)
3 cubes **Ice**

Juicy Instructions

Juice all the fruits and vegetables, then either pour the *extracted juice* into the blender with ice and blend or simply add ice to a glass and pour over.

The Clever Stuff!

When I talk about juicing I always stress the importance of variety. It's important that we use a wide variety of fruits and vegetables in a wide spectrum of colours. This isn't because they look pretty! It's so we can reap the benefits of the unique phyotochemical combinations exclusive to each ingredient. Phytochemicals, simply put, are protective plant chemicals that have an effect on human health by helping to fight or prevent disease. Some more commonly known phytochemicals are flavonoids, carotenoids, limonene and lycopene (to name a few!). A study in the *British Medical Journal* in 2013 found that simply prescribing one apple a day to everyone over the age of 50 would prevent or delay 8,500 vascular deaths, such as heart attacks and strokes, every year in the UK. The effects of this were deemed similar to the effects of prescribing a statin for everyone over 50 (if not already on them). So it seems an apple a day...could keep the heart attack away!

RED CABBAGE is a cruciferous vegetable. A review of research published in the October 1996 issue of the *Journal of the American Dietetic Association* showed that 70 per cent or more of the studies found a link between cruciferous vegetables and protection against cancer. So if you aren't a lover of veg and can't eat them, that's why we drink them! Other cruciferous vegetables include broccoli, cauliflower, Brussels sprouts and kale.

TOMATOES are packed full of antioxidants, lycopene being the most well known. Lycopene is the phytochemical that gives tomatoes their fiery red colour and has also been largely associated with the prevention of some cancers.

CHLOROPHYLL CLEANSER

Makes a showing on days 2, 10, 16 and 24

Chlorophyll is trapped sunlight energy in plants, so if you think about it, a glass of fruit and vegetable juices is the nearest we will ever get to drinking sunshine! Freshly extracted apple, succulent pear combined with the subtle flavours of cucumber, celery and broccoli; the darkest, deepest greens of spinach, kale and a hint of lime.

This delicious glass of sunlight is packed with chlorophyll so you'll be beaming for the rest of the day.

Juicy Ingredients

1 **Apple** (Golden Delicious or Gala)
1 **Pear** (any hard variety)
¼ medium **Cucumber**
½ **Lime** (with rind on)
1 stick **Celery**
1 large handful **Spinach**
3 cm **Broccoli** stem
1 large handful **Kale**
3 cubes **Ice**

Juicy Instructions

Simply juice everything, pour over ice and enjoy!

The Clever Stuff!

Chlorophyll is the molecule in plants that gives them their green colour. It is responsible for facilitating one of the most important processes on earth, that of turning the energy from sunlight, water and carbon monoxide into glucose. Humans and animals depend on plants as their primary food source, with many wild animals living exclusively on vegetation in a state of optimum health, which in itself, without any clinical trials, is ample evidence to support the power of consuming green plant life.

As well as being rich in chlorophyll, **SPINACH** is well known for its iron content. Iron plays a central role in the function of red blood cells that help in transporting oxygen around the body, in energy production and DNA synthesis.

KALE, like spinach, is a versatile leafy green that can be easily disguised in most fruit and veggie blends to up the ante of nutrition. It contains high levels of lutein, an antioxidant which boosts eye health and can help to protect against age related macular degeneration. Because of its high vitamin K content, consuming kale on a regular basis can help with the maintenance of healthy bones as well as with blood clotting.

DIGESTIVE AID

Makes a showing on days 3, 9, 17 and 23

We all need a bit of help sometimes, even our digestive systems! We put it through a lot on a daily basis, often by feasting on the wrong foods, leaving our poor digestive systems to deal with the consequences. The light and relieving juices of crisp apples and carrots, soothing celery, fragrant fennel and the warmth of ginger will calm and soothe your system and give it that well deserved rest and added TLC.

Juicy Ingredients
2 **Apples** (Golden Delicious or Gala)
2 large **Carrot** (remove hard end)
1 stick **Celery**
3 cm **Fennel**
3 cm **Ginger**
3 cubes **Ice**

Juicy Instructions
Simply juice the lot and either pour the into a blender /booster with ice and blend or simply add ice to a glass and pour over.

The Clever Stuff!

Juicing helps to give our digestive system a well-deserved break. Nothing takes up more energy in the body than digestion, so it's important we consume things that are quickly and easily digested. Fresh fruits and vegetables juices are virtually pre-digested.

FENNEL is an excellent source of vitamin C, which neutralizes free radicals that could otherwise cause cellular damage, resulting in pain and disease. It is also a good source of potassium, a vital mineral that is crucial in reducing high blood pressure and thus preventing heart disease and strokes. Fennel has many soothing and therapeutic properties, so it helpful in relieving the symptoms associated with digestive discomfort, including bloating. In fact, it is widely used as an antispasmodic for IBS, because the essential oils contained in fennel help to relax the walls of the gut. Fennel has also been said to release endorphins into the bloodstream. Endorphins are 'feel good chemicals that help in creating a mood of euphoria and are thought to give relief to symptoms of depression and anxiety.

GINGER ROOT (aka zingiber officinale), although considered quite fiery, can also be very warming and settling. Not only can it help with problems such as flatulence, but it also soothes the intestinal tract and helps to stimulate the breakdown of food particles.

ENERGY EXPLOSION

Makes a showing on days 7, 14, 21 and 28

For the times when you just need that little extra...kick up the backside! Your body is going to love this energy-enriched glass of goodness. Bring on the juicy high, which should be very apparent by day seven. Made with pineapple, which creates such sweet, smooth and creamy base, this really is a hard one to beat.

Juicy Ingredients
¼ medium **Pineapple**
1 **Apple** (Golden Delicious or Gala)
2 medium **Carrot**
1 handful **Spinach**
1 handful **Kale**
3 cm **Broccoli** stem
¼ **Lemon** (rind on, wax free)
3 cubes **Ice**

Juicy Instructions
Simply juice the 'hopping pot', that's Cockney rhyming slang for 'the lot'! Pour over ice and enjoy.

The Clever Stuff!

Kale, broccoli and spinach are superb sources of chlorophyll, which is molecularly the same as haemoglobin in the blood except for one central element (iron vs. magnesium). This extraordinary similarity means chlorophyll delivers a continuous energy transfusion into the bloodstream replenishing and increasing red blood cell count, resulting in an increased ability of the red blood cells to carry oxygen. It is an amazing blood cleanser, blood builder and energy supplier. Vegetables contain a high percentage of carbohydrates, your body's primary energy source, whilst the natural sugars in fruits help to boost energy levels.

KALE, actually has more vitamin C than an orange, – who knew! This modest green leafy veg also contains approximately twice your recommended daily intake of vitamin A and seven times the recommended amount of vitamin K. Kale is also a good source of B-complex vitamins, which help extract energy from nutrients. We really have covered all bases in this juice, kale AND spinach.

SPINACH is rich in iron which is an important in the process of energy production in the body. It contains far more than the suggested daily intake of vitamins A and K and nearly all the folic acid and manganese required. It's full of cancer-fighting antioxidants and also helps with the absorption of calcium.

LEMON helps to give this juice an edge. Lemons are antibacterial, antifungal and anti-inflammatory. They contain limonene, a phytochemical that is found in the peel of citrus fruits, has been said to fight cancer cells and is also used in cleaning and cosmetic products.

THE
VERY
SPECIAL
GUESTS

I have introduced some very 'Special Guests' to the *Super Juice Me! 28-Day Juice Plan* and once you taste these beauties, you'll be extremely pleased I did.

These feature on the evenings of days 6 and 7. The vast majority of people will be starting the plan on a Monday, so the 'special guests' have been designed to be a much-welcomed companion for Saturday and Sunday evenings.

All of the specials are made using just a blender (booster), so are quick and easy to make. They also require fresh, raw, protein-rich almond milk, which, you'll be pleased to know, is very easy to make. You'll find all the instructions on page 237. Or you can see me making it on the app.

The almonds will need soaking overnight, so please make a note of this for the evenings of days 5, 12, 19 and 26. If you cannot consume almonds, then alternatives to this are other nut milks, rice milk, soya milk, or you can simply make that day's morning smoothie instead.

HOW TO MAKE ALMOND MILK

Almond skin contains an enzyme inhibitor that protects the almond. For better nutrient bioavailability and absorption the almonds should be soaked overnight.

Ideally soak the almonds on day 5 and make the almond milk required for both days 6 and 7 on day 6.

1 handful Raw Almonds
500 ml Filtered water

The day before

Put the almonds in a bowl and cover with water (this does not need to be filtered water) and leave for at least 8 hours if possible.

The day

Take the soaked almonds and discard the water. Place the soaked almonds in the blender and add the filtered water. Blend for a full minute. Pour the liquid through a sieve, discard the residue nuts and you now have 'almond milk'. This can be stored in the fridge and is best used within 24–48 hours.

---

*   As an alternative to raw almond milk you can use other nut milks, rice milk or soya milk

TAHINI COCOA BEANEY

Makes a showing on days 6 and 20

Your first 'special guest' of the week – and after this, you can never say I am anything other than good to you! Prepare to be impressed. Not only will this smoothie taste like the best chocolate milkshake ever, it is also one of the healthiest. Blending banana with almond milk just creates this beautiful creamy base, complemented by the bitterness from the cocoa, the smooth and silky tones of the tahini and sweetened naturally with a dash of honey. Savour every mouthful.

The 'Special' Ingredients
1 medium **Banana**
1 teaspoon **Raw Cocoa Powder** *
1 teaspoon **Tahini Paste**
1 teaspoon **Manuka Honey**
500 ml **Raw Almond Milk** **
2 cubes **Ice**

The 'Special' Instructions
In the blender put the banana, cocoa, tahini, honey and ice. Pour in the raw almond milk up to the 500 ml line and blend until smooth.

* Available from all good health stores.

** Please refer to recipe on page 237

The Clever Stuff!

Pure cocoa powder is far removed from the sickly sweet, over-processed sugar powder that most people know. Raw cocoa is a rich source of antioxidant goodness. It also contains the substance phenethylamine, a neurotransmitter found in the brain that acts as a mood elevator and natural antidepressant. Cocoa contains an amino acid called tryptophan that will help with relaxation and in turn better sleep.

TAHINI is packed with a range of B vitamins, essential fatty acids (EFAs) and manganese, which are imperative for the health of the brain and nervous system. In fact research has linked an EFA deficiency with a host of diseases, from skin problems through to Alzheimer's disease. Tahini has 20 per cent complete protein, making it a higher protein source than most nuts.

Did you know that **ALMONDS** are not technically nuts; they are actually the seed of the fruit of the almond tree? Almonds are a super source of vitamin E, Biotin, manganese, calcium, magnesium, potassium, iron, zinc and copper. Most traditional 'nuts' are slightly to moderately acidic, however almonds are alkaline forming, mainly due to the fact that they have the highest concentration of calcium than any other 'nut'. They are also a great source of protein and healthy polyunsaturated and monounsaturated fatty acids. Almonds are therefore a wonderfully nutritious and very beneficial food source.

FOR GOODNESS SHAKE

Makes a showing on days 7 and 21

This 'Special Guest' has it all; juicy berries, the creamy blend of banana, almond milk and...spinach? Yes, you did read it right; this is a fruity shake with a difference! It really is amazing the health you can hide, particularly in a smoothie. Seriously, embrace the unknown; you are going to LOVE it!

The 'Special' Ingredients
1 handful mixed **Berries** (fresh or frozen)
1 medium **Banana**
1 handful of baby leaf **Spinach**
500 ml **Raw Almond Milk***
2 cubes **Ice**

The 'Special' Instructions
In the blender put the berries, banana, spinach and ice. Pour in the raw almond milk up to the 500 ml line and blend until smooth.

* Please refer to recipe on page 237

The Clever Stuff!

This smoothie is a wonderful source of fibre, potassium, zinc, protein, magnesium, selenium, unsaturated 'good' fats, and the list goes on and on. It is very satiating or filling and will provide a good gradual release of energy whilst protecting the cardiovascular system and helping to reduce bad cholesterol.

MIXED BERRIES are bursting with antioxidants those fantastic little super nutrients that fight free radical damage that can otherwise harm cells. Remember, you can use fresh or frozen berries. If you use frozen berries, you won't need the ice. Happy days!

Throwing a handful of spinach into the blender is a really neat way of increasing the nutritional impact of any smoothie. Interestingly the impact on the taste of the smoothie is so minor you will barely notice it. This is a really useful way of nutritionally 'beefing' up a smoothie for your little loved ones. You don't even need to mention the addition of the spinach in the recipe, its what's uncommonly known as a little green lie!

SPIRULINA PROTEIN POWER SHAKE

Makes a showing on days 13 and 27.

This shake is a real protein powerhouse that will instantly satiate your appetite and give you a powerful punch of protein. This might seem like an unusual combination of ingredients, but it works perfectly to provide a delicate, creamy smoothie balanced beautifully with a shot of protein rich spirulina.

The 'Special' Ingredients
1 medium **Banana**
1 level teaspoon **Spirulina**
500 ml **Raw Almond Milk***
2 cubes **Ice**

The 'Special' Instructions
In the blender put the banana, spirulina and ice. Pour in the raw almond milk up to the 500 ml line and blend until smooth.

* Please refer to recipe on page 237

The Clever Stuff!

This simple recipe will surprise you, as the combination of these three ingredients tastes utterly divine. On a nutritional level the spirulina seriously enhances this smoothie.

SPIRULINA is a true superfood that provides an excellent source of protein, vitamins and minerals. Protein is not only needed for muscles but for other functions we often don't think of, such as the production of infection-fighting antibodies. Studies have shown that spirulina can help increase production of these antibodies and this is why it is heralded as such an excellent immune booster.

BANANAS, rather surprisingly, are over 70 per cent water, so, just like all their other fruit and vegetable friends, bananas are great for hydration. They contain sucrose, fructose and glucose, which provide an instant energy boost as well as a sustained and controlled release of blood sugar.

ALMOND MILK provides a great source of calcium and vitamin D and these two nutrients work synergistically to support healthy bones and teeth and thus reduces your risk of developing arthritis and osteoporosis.

SWEET VANILLA SHAKE

Makes a showing on days 14 and 28.

It is just RIDICULOUS how good this tastes! It's like your favourite vanilla milkshake but healthy! It really is everything you imagine it to be a sweet, satiating and stupidly scrumptious.

The 'Special' Ingredients
1 medium **Banana**
1 teaspoon **Manuka Honey**
1 pod or 1 teaspoon of extract **Vanilla** (extract or beans from pod)
500 ml **Raw Almond Milk***
2 cubes **Ice**

The 'Special' Instructions
In the blender put the banana, honey, vanilla beans or extract and ice. Pour in the raw almond milk up to the 500 ml line and blend until smooth.

* Please refer to recipe on page 237

The Clever Stuff!

One of the reasons this smoothie tastes so divine is because of the rich vanilla bean flavour. The chances are the pods you are using were grown in Madagascar, Indonesia, Puerto Rica or the West Indies. So enjoy this drink that originated in paradise simply because it tastes so sublime and not because it is the most nutritious smoothie on the plan. Vanilla is an aromatic spice that is a source of antioxidants and is also believed to benefit the nervous system. Honey soothes sore throats and kills bacteria that cause infection and is widely used as a natural sweetener.

The banana provides the smooth, creamy flavour as well as thickening this smoothie so it really feels satiating. Despite what some people believe, bananas contain no fat or cholesterol, they are however a great source of natural carbohydrates and natural sugar as well as fibre and potassium. They are great for slow release energy, regulating blood sugar levels and aiding the function of the heart and other muscles.

Because 'home-made, raw' almond milk is not cooked or processed, it is abundant in vitamins, minerals and enzymes. On top of that it is a wonderful source of protein and contains good fats, but unlike real milk, contains no cholesterol, saturated fats, lactose or gluten. Almond milk really is the new 'black' and hopefully after this plan it will become a nutritious and delicious staple in your diet.

HUNGER SOS!

No recipes needed for this as, nature, Juice Master, or another good natural energy bar company will have done then work for you!

THE OPTIONS:

- 1 x small banana (Fairtrade)

- 1 x medium avocado

- Juice In A Bar (veggie or fruit versions)

- Simply Nude

PLEASE NOTE:

As per the guidelines set out in 'Top Ten Tips For Juicy Success' (page 145) only *one* Hunger SOS is available to you each day and there's no 'rollover' if you don't use one! I would advise only using the SOS as just that, a genuine SOS, and I would also advise not having any SOS until after the first 7 days, where possible.

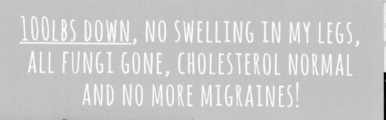

100LBS DOWN, NO SWELLING IN MY LEGS, ALL FUNGI GONE, CHOLESTEROL NORMAL AND NO MORE MIGRAINES!

Chris Stewart

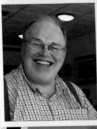

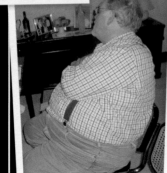

- BEFORE -

- AFTER -

"I have definitely Super Juiced myself!
My list of improvements are endless from
energy, mental clarity, normal blood
pressure, cholesterol – all thanks to juicing."

50.7LBS LOST AND I FEEL SO ENERGIZED AND HEALTHY

Aliya Kassam

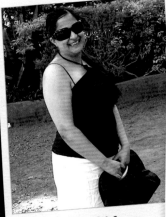

- BEFORE -

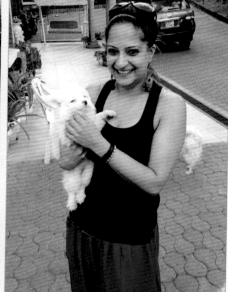

- AFTER -

"Who wouldn't want to try this?
It's the easiest and healthiest
way to lose weight."

Thanks to juicing
I have cured my Type 2 diabetes

Jason Levy

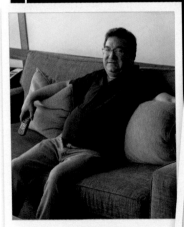

- BEFORE -

"I feel I have been given a second chance."

- AFTER -

"Since I have Super Juiced! myself I am celebrating one of the happiest days of my life. I no longer need to be on medication. I have cured my type 2 diabetes. My blood pressure is healthy, my cholesterol is normal. All my blood sugars are perfect."

Juicing gave me a second chance...
I lost 270 pounds

Kitten Barbosa

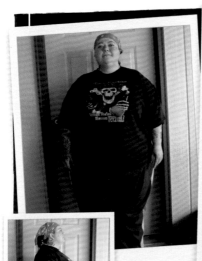

- BEFORE -

- AFTER -

"Juicing has done so much for me. No
more headaches, no more crutches.
My leg is normal, my skin cleared up,
no more mood swings. I can now walk
without struggling for breath."

100LBS LIGHTER
I have been Super Juiced!

Andrew Tubbs

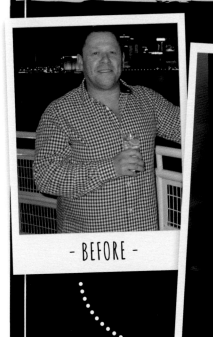

- BEFORE -

- AFTER -

"I turned 50 this year and I feel like I am in my twenties. All my friends and family now juice thanks to Jason."

ALL MY HEALTH PROBLEMS HAVE VANISHED!

Kelly Gill

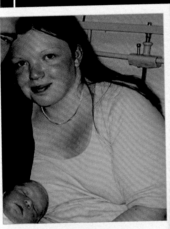

- BEFORE -

"I'M HAPPIER, HEALTHIER AND FINALLY IN CONTROL."

- AFTER -

"For years I have been hiding at home shackled by fatigue and anxiety. Epileptic seizures, IBS and eczema... Now thanks to juicing I have dropped 5 dress sizes, I haven't had a single seizure, I am off all medication which I have been taking since the age of 9! And my eczema has gone!"

105LBS LOST AND I HAVE SOOO MUCH MORE CONFIDENCE IN MYSELF

Jason Bray

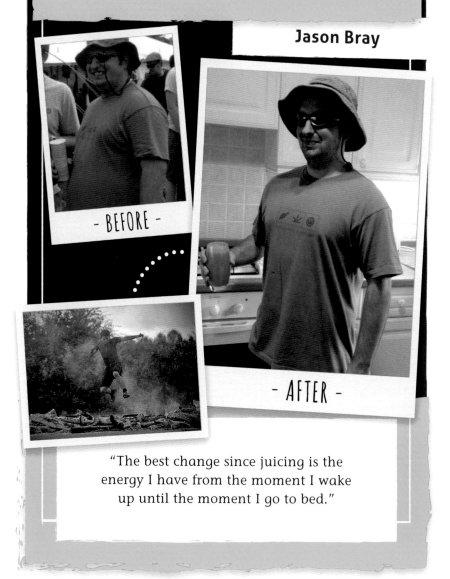

- BEFORE -

- AFTER -

"The best change since juicing is the energy I have from the moment I wake up until the moment I go to bed."

I'VE <u>LOST 123LBS</u>, STOPPED SMOKING AND THINK SO MUCH MORE CLEARLY

Brendan Turner

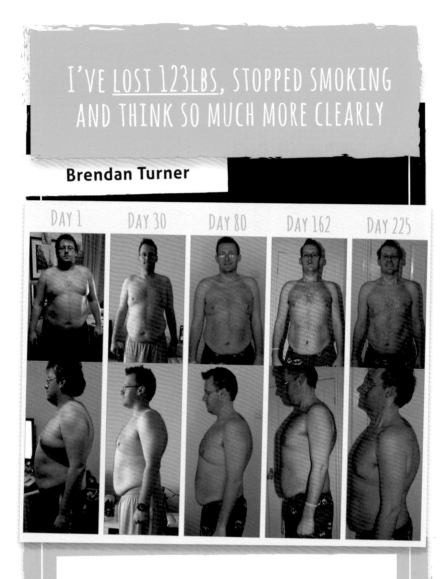

DAY 1   DAY 30   DAY 80   DAY 162   DAY 225

"I no longer suffer from sleep apnea,
my skin and hair condition have improved.
I have more energy plus, I now crave fresh
healthy raw vegetables and salads."

MORE ENERGY, NO MORE ASTHMA, SLEEPING BETTER AND OVERALL 35LBS GONE NOT BAD AT <u>80 YEARS OF AGE!</u>

Pauline Doran

"I DON'T FEEL SO OLD NOW."

- FEELING GREAT AT 80! -

"My doctor told me that I have saved the NHS thousands of pound as I didn't need the knee re-placement - all thanks to juicing. I used to have lots of chest infections or Bronchitis, but I haven't had even a sniffley cold for over 18 months."

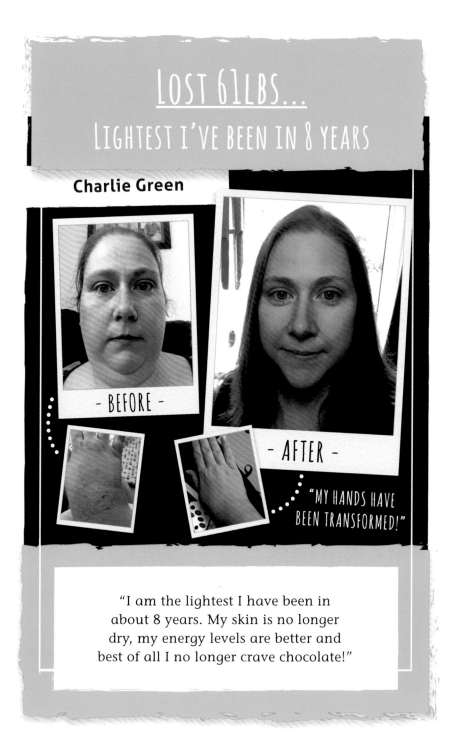

Lost 61lbs...

Lightest i've been in 8 years

Charlie Green

- BEFORE -

- AFTER -

"MY HANDS HAVE BEEN TRANSFORMED!"

"I am the lightest I have been in about 8 years. My skin is no longer dry, my energy levels are better and best of all I no longer crave chocolate!"

AMAZING! PSORIASIS CLEARED, ECZEMA CLEARED, 55LBS WEIGHT LOST

Hanna Sillitoe

- BEFORE -

"THERE ARE SO MANY THINGS THAT CAN BENEFIT FROM A PROGRAMME THAT STARTS BY 'CURING' YOU FROM THE INSIDE NOT THE OUTSIDE"

- AFTER -

"Juicing cured my Psoriasis something I'd tried for over twenty years to heal using conventional medicine, and didn't work. As far-fetched and kooky as it sounds, that leafy, vegetable drink was the catalyst for a huge transformation in my skin, my body and my mind."

35LBS LIGHTER...
BLOOD PRESSURE HAS DROPPED
FROM 134/78 to 110/74

Marc Mulligan

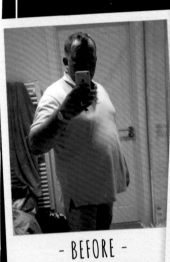

- BEFORE -

- AFTER -

"The health benefits are endless. I will be juicing for life. Since I have been super juiced the stock market price for Rennie has hit an all time low due to the lack of revenue from me!"

35LBS LIGHTER AND FEELING ABSOLUTELY FULL OF ENERGY

Rachel Johnson

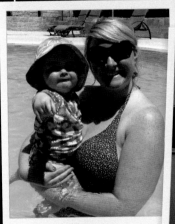

- BEFORE -

- AFTER -

"Doing the juice programme has shown me that you really can achieve anything you put your mind to. I chose to be healthier, for my skin to glow and for people to tell me I look the best I've looked in years. Honestly – I could not be happier."

JUICING MADE ME <u>LOSE 56LBS</u>

Ama Uzowuru

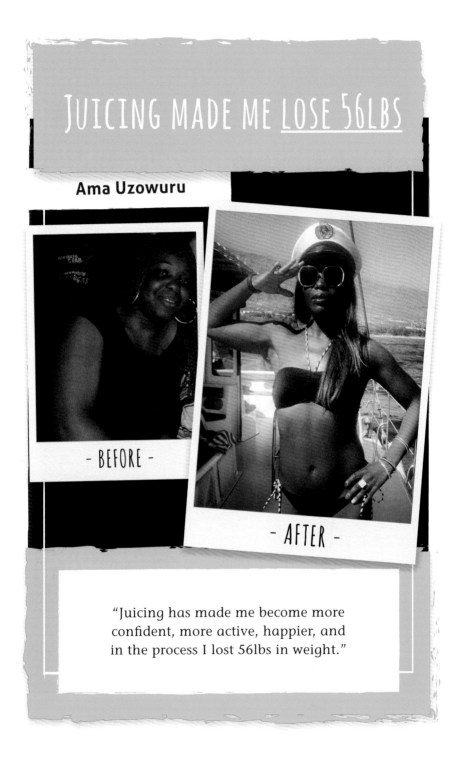

- BEFORE -

- AFTER -

"Juicing has made me become more confident, more active, happier, and in the process I lost 56lbs in weight."

THANKS TO JUICING I HAVE LOST AND I no longer have diabetes

Anthony Jones

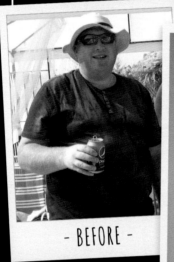

- BEFORE -

"I AM ALIVE AND LIVING AND FEELING GREAT."

- AFTER -

"Today, thanks to juicing, I am 105lbs lighter, no longer have diabetes, go to the gym at least 3 day a week, cycle 20 miles a week and walk my dog 2-4 miles every day."

Eczema gone 22lbs lost!

Christine Bean

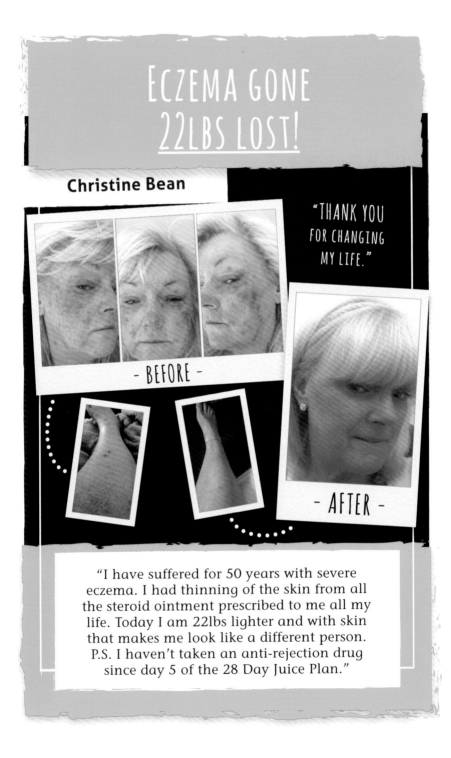

"THANK YOU FOR CHANGING MY LIFE."

- BEFORE -

- AFTER -

"I have suffered for 50 years with severe eczema. I had thinning of the skin from all the steroid ointment prescribed to me all my life. Today I am 22lbs lighter and with skin that makes me look like a different person. P.S. I haven't taken an anti-rejection drug since day 5 of the 28 Day Juice Plan."

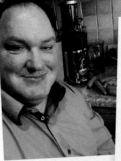

I WAS MORBIDLY OBESE, HAD BLOOD PRESSURE AND MY LIVER WAS NOT IN GOOD SHAPE.... JUICING HAS TURNED ALL OF THIS AROUND

Adam Harding-Jones

- BEFORE -

- AFTER -

"Thanks to Jason's motivation and juice I have just completed a 50 mile bike event and now planning my 100 mile event. I have also just completed Tough Mudder North West."

I HAVE LOST 140LBS THANKS TO JUICING

David Hochmuth

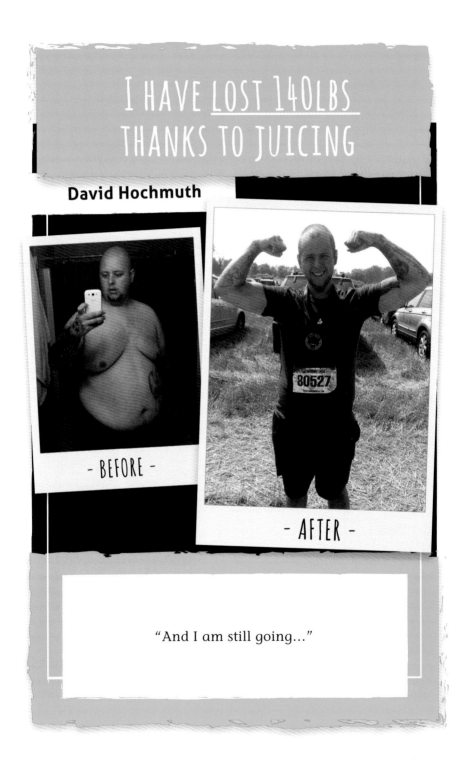

- BEFORE -

- AFTER -

"And I am still going…"

I HAVE <u>LOST 33POUNDS</u>
I FEEL INCREDIBLE, LIKE I CAN TAKE ON ANY CHALLENGE LIFE THROWS AT ME!

Michelle Thomas

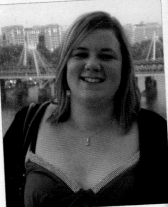

- BEFORE -

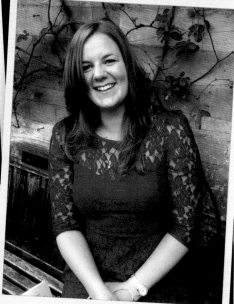

- AFTER -

"I have just completed the 28 day programme and I am officially a Super Juicer! It was not as difficult as I had led myself to think it would be – I didn't really miss eating food, I wasn't hungry for the most part and didn't have any cravings for junk etc."

Hannah Busby

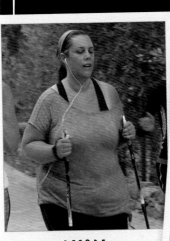

- BEFORE -

- AFTER -

"I have completely changed my mindset
towards food, exercise and myself.
I have so much more energy and
I think much more clearly."

MY SUPER JUICE ME! JOURNAL

Never underestimate the power of writing things down

13

KEEP A JOURNAL

Welcome to the start of what I hope to be a genuine life-changing experience for you. Many people find it incredibly valuable to keep a journal of their experience, so I have included this space in the book so you can do just that. I believe that keeping your journal within the book is more effective than keeping it elsewhere. This is because you will inevitably want to keep your journal with you and you will always have access to the information in this book for the whole 28 days, should you need to reference it. Please don't underestimate the power of keeping a journal or of returning to certain chapters of the book in order to keep you on track.

GET YOUR BODY STATS

It is also extremely important to get all of your body stats done just before you start. The more you can get the better, including things like **cholesterol, blood sugars, blood-pressure, weight, body measurements,** and so on. If you don't do this, you will never truly know just how far you have travelled and just how potentially effective this plan is. I would also advise good 'before-and-after' photos. It is also good to note down what drugs you are on now, the doses you are on, and how things have changed by the end. Please remember to keep a note of any time you see your doctor throughout this process, and if you are able to reduce your intake of any medical drugs you may be on.

Please remember:

I do not advise you come off any drugs until you first consult your doctor

I would also like you to share your stats with us once you are 'Super Juiced!' Please send an email with your stats, your experience, your before-and-after pictures and so on, with the heading 'I've Been Super Juiced', to results@superjuiceme. com. I am looking to compile as many before-and-after stats as possible in order to do what I can to convince the NHS (National Health Service in the UK) that they need to start looking at juice-based therapy as a genuine alternative to drug-based medicine. We need to move away from the 'a pill for every ill and an ill for pill' approach for everything. I honestly believe this approach has the potential to help restore good health in many, whilst saving the NHS millions of £s. As already mentioned in this book, but worth repeating here, Roger Gale, who appeared in the movie Super Juice Me!, worked out that the NHS had saved over £100,000 on him alone. One year on (as I write this book), Roger is still drug free and costing the NHS ABSOLUTELY NOTHING! Many people are doing this for weight loss, so it's also worth pointing out that, at time of writing this book, the average gastric bypass operation costs between £8,000 and £10,000 – just slightly more than some fresh fruit and veg and a juicer! The more evidence we can present the more likely we are to see a breakthrough in this area, and juice therapy may just become part of the tool-kit doctors use to treat people.

DON'T BE A WEIGHT WATCHER!

On a final note before you start, please also refrain from weighing yourself every day. Weight fluctuates and you should weigh yourself only after the first week, and then again at the end. It's always tempting to jump on the scales every two minutes, but it won't serve you, and it can have the opposite effect.

STARTING BODY STATS

Weight	
Height	
Waist	
Chest	
Hips	
Body Fat %	
Cholesterol	
Blood Pressure	
Blood Sugars	
General Mood	
Energy Levels	
Conditions/ Diseases/ Illnesses	
Medical Drugs and Doses	

DAY 1*

'The food you eat can be either the safest & the most powerful form of medicine or the slowest form of poison.'
Anne Wigmore

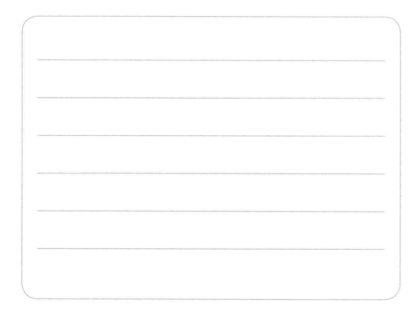

* If you have the app (or DVD) please make a point of watching the Day 1 video today. Everything you need to know is in this book clearly, so don't worry if you don't have the app. However, never underestimate the power of a little coaching. You are undertaking a big challenge here, one which many would never even attempt, so if you do have the app please watch the video as it can make all the difference.

DAY 2

'Every step toward your dream today
is a step away from your regret tomorrow.'
Dr Steve Maraboli

DAY 3

'Strength does not come from winning. Your struggles
develop your strengths. When you go through hardships
and decide not to surrender, that is strength.'
Arnold Schwarzegger

DAY 4

'I've missed more than 9000 shots in my career. I've lost almost 300 games. 26 times I've been trusted to take the game winning shot and missed. I've failed over and over and over again in my life. And that is why I succeed.'

Michael Jordan

DAY 5

'The best time to plant a tree was twenty years ago.
The second best time is now.'
Chinese Proverb

DAY 6

'I am not a product of my circumstances.
I am a product of my decisions.'
Stephen Covey

DAY 7

'Whether you think you can or you
think you can't, you're right.'
Henry Ford

DAY 8*

'There is only one way to avoid criticism: do nothing,
say nothing, and be nothing.'
Aristotle

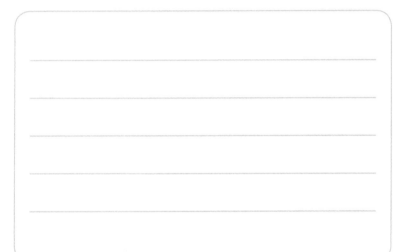

* It's the start of week two! Firstly, you're a quarter of the way through, and if all is going to plan, you should have already dropped some weight and come out of the 'fog'. There will still be highs and lows throughout the 28 days, but you should have a decent amount of momentum now. If you have the app, don't forget the to watch the week 2 video today. I get emails every day from people who have done the plan, and most say they couldn't have done it without the added support of the coaching on the app. Please, if you have it, watch the videos.

DAY 9

'Believe you can and you're halfway there.'
Theodore Roosevelt

DAY 10

'Everything you've ever wanted is on the other side of fear.'
George Adair

DAY 11

'When I was 5 years old, my mother always told me that happiness was the key to life. When I went to school, they asked me what I wanted to be when I grew up. I wrote down 'happy'. They told me I didn't understand the assignment, and I told them they didn't understand life.'

John Lennon

DAY 12

'Happiness is not something ready-made.
It comes from your own actions.'
Dalai Lama

DAY 13

'Challenges are what make life interesting and
overcoming them is what makes life meaningful.'
Joshua J. Marine

DAY 14

'Limitations live only in our minds. But if we use our imaginations, our possibilities become limitless.'
Jamie Paolinetti

DAY 15*

'You'll have bad times but it'll always wake you up to the good stuff you weren't paying attention to.'
Robin Williams in *Good Will Hunting*

* Start of week 3 and, if you are going to struggle at all, then week 3 is where it hits people the most. It's like running a marathon or writing a book. Everyone is there with you at the start and also the end, but the middle is where it's a test of human character. On the upside, you are already half-way through, and if you've come this far and feel this good already, imagine how good you'll be feeling at the end. Once again, if you have the app make a point of watching the week 3 video. I would say it is one of the most important ones.

DAY 16

'If you can dream it, you can achieve it.'
Zig Ziglar

DAY 17

'When you get into a tight place and everything goes
against you, till it seems you could not hang on a minute
longer, never give up then, for that is just the place and
time that the tide will turn.'
Harriet Beecher Stowe

DAY 18

'Knowing is not enough; we must apply.
Willing is not enough; we must do.'
Johann Wolfgang von Goethe

DAY 19

'Life has no smooth road for any of us; and in the bracing
atmosphere of a high aim the very roughness stimulates the
climber to steadier steps, till the legend, over steep ways to
the stars, fulfills itself.'
W. C. Doane

DAY 20

'The difference between a successful person and others is
not a lack of strength, not a lack of knowledge,
but rather a lack in will.'
Vince Lombardi

DAY 21

'Success is to be measured not so much by the position that one has reached in life as by the obstacles which he has overcome while trying to succeed.'
Booker T. Washington

DAY 22 *

Some people want it to happen, some wish it would
happen, others make it happen!

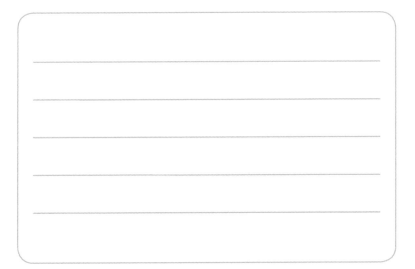

* You are well and truly on the home straight, three weeks
in the bag and just one to go! Congratulations on what you
have achieved this far. If you have the app, watch the video
for week 3 to make sure the final week is as easy as possible.
I have also recorded an SOS video for each week and you
may well have watched them over the past three weeks. I
debated whether to do one for the final week. Surely you
wouldn't throw in the towel now? In the end I decided to
record one, if you need it, it's there.

DAY 23

'Tough times never last, but tough people do.'
Dr. Robert Schuller

DAY 24

'Don't count the days, make the days count.'
Muhammad Ali

DAY 25

'The difference between ordinary and
extraordinary is that little extra.'
Jimmy Johnson

DAY 26

'It is never too late to be what you might have been.'
George Eliot

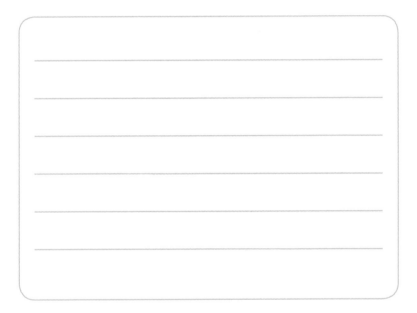

* If you have the app (or DVD), don't forget to watch the day 26 video. It explains exactly what options are open to you after the *28-Day Super Juice Me! Challenge*. I have also explained it in the SUPER FOOD ME! chapter in this book (page 295), but I feel the video on the app or DVD has more clout!

DAY 27

'Obsessed is just a word the lazy use
to describe the dedicated.'
Russell Warren

DAY 28

FINAL DAY
CONGRATULATIONS!

'There are no short cuts to any place worth going.'
Beverly Sills

DAY 29 – results day

Weight	
Height	
Waist	
Chest	
Hips	
Body Fat %	
Cholesterol	
Blood Pressure	
Blood Sugars	
General Mood	
Energy Levels	
Conditions/ Diseases/ Illnesses	
Medical Drugs and Doses	

CONGRATULATIONS

YOU'VE BEEN

SUPER JUICED!

SO WHAT NEXT?

Your next move is to make sure you don't undo all you have achieved on the Super Juice Me! 28-Day Juice Challenge

14

Before we get onto what to do next, I would like to be one of the first to congratulate you on successfully completing the *Super Juice Me! 28-Day Juice Challenge*. Many people are very good at talking about making a change, but few actually end up taking action. You not only declared to the world you were starting this journey, but you have done whatever it has taken to complete it. Having personally done the Super Juice Me! *28-Day Juice Challenge* on more than one occasion, I am fully aware of the journey you have been on and I have the upmost respect for you.

If you are like the vast majority of people who reach this stage, you should be feeling a damned sight better than when you started. If you have time, I really would love to know your before-and-after story, including pictures and stats, if possible, to results@superjuiceme.com. Nothing helps to inspire others more than *real* stories from *real* people. Your story could just tip the balance for someone who is currently *thinking* about doing something about their health and weight into *actually* doing something about it. The more genuine results we get in, the more we can help to convince the medical community that this is a drug free, alternative option which is worth looking at. It is my aim to get juicing into hospitals, but that will only happen by convincing politicians, and *that* will only happen if we have enough evidence to support it. So if you have had great results, I would appreciate it if you could take time to send them in. Thank you in advance for taking the time to do this and for helping to make a difference.

I sincerely hope that whatever health issue that led you to embark on the *Super Juice Me! 28-Day Juice Challenge* has improved to some extent. At the very start of this book I mentioned that not every health condition will improve within the 28 days, or, perhaps, at all. What I made a point of saying over and over again was that the *vast majority* of people experience a very positive response to the *Super Juice Me!* plan. I hope you have been one of them.

One thing is for sure, unlike many medical drugs the pure juice which flows freely inside every single fruit and vegetable designed for humankind, will not have done any harm. What is also clear is that if you were doing this for weight loss, there is no question but that you will have had enormous success in that area in a relatively short space of time. I have seen people drop as much as 40lbs during the *Super Juice Me!* month alone. Please let me know if you beat this record!

I say 'during the *Super Juice Me!* month alone', because for many this is just the start, and what you do immediately after Super Juicing yourself, is just as important as, if not more important than, the *Super Juice Me!* month itself.

One cannot and should not live on juice alone forever – we have teeth and a digestive system for a reason!

Remember, living on nothing but juice for 28 days is *not* a normal thing to do, but then living on chips, cake, chocolate, alcohol and fast food in the absence of fresh produce is also not normal. At times we have to do that which appears abnormal simply in order to try and counter the abnormalities which have occurred from a *very* abnormal diet.

Now that you have done the *28-Day Super Juice Me! Challenge*, the last thing you want to do is go straight back to your old abnormal diet and end up in exactly the same place you were in before you started. This is where many who criticize the *Super Juice Me!* plan get it wrong. (A certain TV doctor in the UK springs to mind!) They wrongly say that as soon as a person goes back to eating normally they will gain all the weight back again.

My reply is this. First, not everyone does the *28-Day Super Juice Me! Challenge* for weight loss; many do it for health reasons. Secondly, it's all down to our understanding of the word 'normal' here. If the critics' 'normal' diet was one of chips, chocolate, fast food, alcohol and the like and they go back to that 'normal', then, yes, they will indeed get fat and sick again. This happens not because of the juice, but because of the over-consumption of refined fat, salt and sugar! It is claimed that it's a metabolism thing. It is claimed that because you've been on nothing but juice your metabolism would have gone down, and the second you start to eat 'normally' again, you'll pile on the pounds (or kilos for my European readers). This is, for want of a better expression, total bull! If you eat salads, lean proteins, fresh fruit and skip the refined fat, salt and sugar, then not only will you maintain your weight loss, but the body will also continue to lose more, if it needs to, and remain healthy. If you think, 'Yeah, I've done the challenge', and celebrate by shovelling shed-loads of crap down your throat, guess what? You'll soon be back where you started. Not because there was a change in your metabolism caused by the juice plan, or because the *Super Juice Me!* plan didn't work for you, but because you've gone back to what caused the problem in the first place. If it caused it once, it will cause it again! If you go back to your old ways, it is your responsibility; it is not because *Super Juice Me!* failed you, but because you failed it!

DON'T 'YES BUT...' YOUR WAY BACK TO OBESITY AND ILL HEALTH

The 28-Day Juice Plan is designed to be the ultimate kick-*start*, not kick-end. So many people, when they finish a 'diet' of any kind, celebrate by eating the same crap that got them into the fat and ill world in the first place. They then wonder why they end up back where they started and, almost without fail, blame the diet or something else for getting them back to square one – or, rather, *round* one!

As I mentioned in the DITCH THE EXCUSES chapter, I have heard not only just about every excuse under the sun as to why people never even start to do anything about their weight and health, but I have also heard every excuse in the book as to why they go back to their old ways, even if they do lose weight and gain better health. None of the excuses ever really hold water, but some hold less than others.

Here's what I can only describe as the most stupid and nonsensical 'YES, BUT…' excuse I have ever heard as to why someone went back to their old behaviour. I want to add it here so that you never ever feel that anything like this is in any way a valid excuse for returning to the land of the fat and sick. I heard it years ago when I was running an Allen Carr Stop Smoking clinic in Birmingham. Although it relates to smoking, it beautifully illustrates the madness of this type of excuse. At the time there was a very popular morning show on Virgin radio, 'The Chris Evans Show', with Chris and a few co-presenters bringing some life to the nation's weekday mornings. One morning they were all talking about smoking and I heard one of the co-presenters say, and I quote, 'I heard Allen Carr is smoking again'. Now I was running an Allen Carr Stop Smoking clinic, so this was not exactly great press. At the clinic we offered a money-back guarantee, if you didn't stop smoking. In order to get your money back, you had to fulfil the terms of that guarantee, one of which was that you had to attend two refresher sessions within three months, if the first hadn't quite done the trick.

The same day as the co-presenter's announcement to the world that Allen was smoking again, I received a call from a woman who had attended the clinic and told me, in no uncertain terms, 'I WANT MY MONEY BACK'. I looked for her appointment card (seems odd now that we didn't have a computer or email) and noticed she had attended the clinic some eight months prior. I explained she was out of the three months and asked if she had started within three months of her session with us. She said she'd left the clinic and had not smoked until today. She explained she had found it easy and not really struggled. I asked, 'What on earth made you start smoking today?' She replied, 'because I heard on the radio this morning that Allen Carr was smoking again.' I honestly thought I was hearing things, but she was 100 per cent serious, and she's far from the only one who uses others people's failure to justify their own.

As it turned out Allen hadn't started smoking again and the co-presenter had got her facts wrong, something which later cost Chris Evans £100,000 in court! The point I am making though, is: what does it matter if Allen had picked up a cigarette again? If I were in quicksand and someone helped me out, I wouldn't ever jump back in just because I'd heard that the person who had helped me had gone back in! I wouldn't think for a second that the *method* they'd used to help me get out didn't work just because they'd fallen back in!

This woman's 'YES, BUT…' was to say, 'YES, BUT…Allen's smoking again, so it clearly doesn't work, and it's not my fault I'm smoking again.' This sounds insane when you read it in cold, hard print, but this is not a unique 'YES, BUT…' excuse. I've heard variations on this theme many times, especially when it comes to weight and health. People blame the fact that others fail for their own failure, saying that it doesn't working in the long term, rather than acknowledging that THEY hadn't stuck at it in the long term!

You have just completed the *Super Juice Me! Challenge*, and if you're like most people, you'll be feeling a damned site lighter and healthier than before you started. Now imagine you happily are continuing with a healthy lifestyle and still feel amazing. Imagine you are months down the line and you hear that I, Jason Vale, the juice guy, had stacked a load of weight on again, that my psoriasis had come back, that I was badly asthmatic again, that I had started smoking and drinking again and that I no longer juiced? Would you throw in the juice towel and say, 'Well, clearly it doesn't work. Look at Jason!'? No, of course you wouldn't, because THAT WOULD BE MADNESS! However, if you did ever go back to your old ways, you could always use me as a wonderful 'YES, BUT…' excuse! If I did start to eat rubbish again, started smoking again, got fat and ill again and so on, it doesn't mean that what I teach doesn't work; it means that I'm not doing what I teach! That's my bag, not yours.

YES, BUT WHAT HAPPENED TO THE PEOPLE IN THE FILM?

It would be the same thing if any of the Super Juicers who took part in the film were to ever fall back into their old ways. It's not a valid excuse for *you* to fall back into your old ways. The *Super Juice Me! 28-Day Experiment* was just that, an experiment. It was to see if lifestyle diseases could improve without drug therapy, removing the rubbish coming into the body and replacing the deficiencies with freshly extracted juice. The *Super Juice Me! Experiment* worked, beautifully, as you saw in the film. What the people who took part do afterwards is *their* responsibility and *their* call.

PERSONAL RESPONSIBILITY IS THE KEY TO LIFELONG SUCCESS

If any of them stop doing the plan, that doesn't mean the plan doesn't work; it means they stopped doing the very thing that was working for them. There is no question about it. If any of the Super Juicers started eating nothing but crap again and stopped moving, they would indeed pile the weight back on, they'd get sick and no doubt, they'd be back on the medical pills. I hope this doesn't happen to any of them, but if it does it's because THEY STOPPED DOING WHAT WORKED!

People love any excuse, and if they can use other people's failures as the 'reason' for their failure, they will do so, even if it makes no rational sense at all. However, when everyone is collectively using excuse after excuse to justify their overeating or failure to get off their arses, others around simply nod in agreement. It backs up their excuses too. It's far easier to blame others than it is to take a cold hard look at ourselves. It's much easier to tear down than it is to build up.

Hopefully, if you are like most people, the last thing you'll want to do is to go back to your old 'normal', which in reality was never *normal* at all, as far as your cells were concerned. What most people want to do is to create a new normal for themselves, one that will serve them and one that also takes our being human into account. I have said that living on nothing but juice for 28 days is abnormal; we have only done such a thing to counter the abnormalities which have happened because of our abnormal diet. Equally, I also believe that living on nothing but salad for the rest of your life is also unrealistic and doesn't take into account the human nature of, well, being human! Luckily, the human body has an extremely powerful filtration system and it can handle a certain amount of *anything*, but we need to get the ratio right.

If you are like most people, at the end of the *Super Juice Me! 28-Day Juice Challenge* you'll be craving some solid food. However, if all has gone according to plan it won't be steak and chips, but a large avocado salad or some hot fish on a bed of green leaves.

When it comes to what to do next, there is only one logical place to go. Now that you've done *Super Juice Me!* it's time to…

SUPER FOOD ME!

15

Super Food Me! is a book all unto itself. By the time you read this, it may already be out. People have asked me for years for a full-on 'Jamie Oliver' style healthy food cookbook, and I am finally doing one; *Jason Vale's Low H.I. Cook Book* will be here soon*ish*. However, you don't need it to know what to do after Super Juicing yourself, because I'm going to lay out some very clear guidelines in this chapter.

The term 'superfood' has been overused, but as far as I'm concerned, all fruits, vegetables, nuts, seeds, and lean proteins are superfoods. I honestly believe the term 'superfood' has come about only since the invention, if you will, of non-superfoods, such as refined sugar, refined fats, fast food, chips, cookies, fries and so on. There once was a time, not that long ago in reality, when pretty much all food was what's now termed 'superfood'.

Back in the day, our food wasn't anywhere near as processed and denatured as it is today. High-fructose corn syrup, to give just one example, didn't exist, and most of our food came from the earth and farms, not from a chemical factory. These days you need a degree in chemical science just to read half of the ingredients on most packaged foods, let alone pronounce them. Only a couple of generations past most of the food people ate grew on trees, in the good soil, or was farmed in a 'free range' way. These days food is all about how long can it stay on a supermarket shelf, rather than about whether it holds any genuine nutrition or not, or whether it will actually feed your cells or not. It is also all about addictive chemicals which turn our food into the nicotine of our generation.

In many ways what 'BIG FOOD', if you will, are doing, is far worse than what the tobacco companies did and are still doing today. We need food for our very survival, we clearly don't need nicotine. BIG FOOD manipulate the very thing we need for our survival. They use every trick in the book, from using 'Green' on their labels to dupe us into making an instant subconscious healthy association, to lacing their wares with the perfect combination of refined fat, salt and sugar, designed to trigger a 'bliss point' in our brains so we become addicted. Much of the food industry is no longer a food industry as such, but rather an industry of science, manipulation and addiction. 'Once you pop, you can't stop' applies only to 'food' which has been manipulated in some way to keep you coming back for more. You don't feel the same compulsion with apples! When you eat an apple you don't have an overwhelming compulsion to eat 10 more, but the second you eat a chemically enriched potato chip (crisps to you and me in the UK) you have an instant desire for more.

BIG FOOD is now even more powerful than BIG TOBACCO, and as with anything worth trillions of dollars, it has huge influence over what legislation comes to pass. This is why you soon won't even be able to use the term 'superfood' on food products, as they claim that superfoods don't exist, that all food is good, and no food should be given 'super' status.

I agree that, if you don't have access to any food at all,

then clearly *any* food you *are* able to get hold of is good, even if it's full of refined fat, salt and sugar. If you live in, say, a developing country and are starving, then I believe it could be argued that *all* food is a superfood. However, when you are lucky enough to have a choice over what you eat – I am guessing the vast majority of people reading this book fall into this category – then not all food is the same, and some foods are indeed 'super' by comparison.

And that's the point. These superfoods are super only compared to the *non*-superfoods the vast majority of people in the developed world are consuming on a daily basis. In the wild, animals *only* consume superfoods. All food consumed in the wild is eaten in its natural, 'live' state; animals don't cook their food *ever*. A squirrel, for example, would never describe the nuts it eats as a superfood; to the squirrel it's just food. However, if all the other nuts were covered in fat, salt and sugar and heavily processed, and no longer contained the genuine nutrition of a natural nut, then the natural, unprocessed nut could be defined as 'super'. This is because it will have feeding and healing powers that the heavily processed nuts no longer have.

I agree that the term 'superfood' sounds ridiculous and sounds completely made up in order to sell some Amazonian rainforest berries. I have no doubt some use it for that purpose, but the reason why goji berries, acai berries, blueberries, broccoli, spinach and so on are often refereed to as superfoods is because, compared to the heavily processed crap most people are eating and drinking, they are! It's like the first time I saw Fairtrade bananas. All it did was to draw my attention to the fact that all the rest were in some way unfair.

ALL FRUITS AND VEGETABLES ARE SUPERFOODS

Scurvy killed thousands of people for years, yet a simple lime ended up being the cure. All food designed by nature for our consumption was designed to be both food and medicine. 'Super', I feel, is a fair description for such foods. This is why, now that you've successfully completed the *Super Juice Me! Challenge* it is wise to not undo all of that commitment. Make sure Super Juices and Super Foods continue play a key role in your diet. This doesn't mean being 100 per cent perfect. The perfection game is not one anyone should play; we are all human and should always allow ourselves to be just that from time to time. However, your system is as clean as a whistle at this time, so it is vital not to eat a massive *non*-superfood meal on day 29! You must ease into it. I will outline 10 different ways you can go on from here in the next chapter. You don't have to adhere to any of them. They are just suggestions based on my 15 years of experience in this field. We are all different and we all lead very different lives, so we need to adjust accordingly and do what fits with *our* life, not someone else's. If you have the *Super Juice Me!* app, make a point of watching the final video too.

Before we get onto the top 10 suggestions for after the *Super Juice Me!* plan, I wish to outline two simple concepts. If you adhere to these alone, you'll be flying from here on in.

GO 'NO-LABEL'!

For years I was asked over and over again by people concerned about their health, 'What am I looking for on the label?' It took me many years to realize that the problem was the label itself! As soon as I realized this, whenever people asked me, 'What am I looking for on the label?', I'd simply reply by saying, 'THE LABEL!'

Fruits, vegetables, grains, nuts, seeds and lean proteins don't require a label, and these are the very superfoods we need to be consuming the vast majority of the time, if we are to stay lean and healthy. It's not even something we need a lesson in; we all know *instinctively* what is meant by 'no-label food'. It's the only food *all* wild animals consume and it's the food we would naturally be drawn to if BIG FOOD hadn't manipulated and chemicalized our food. It is also the food that you should be naturally drawn to now that you have 'Super Juiced' yourself. Your system is clean and, like I mentioned, any junk food addiction should have subsided and you should now be naturally craving non-label foods.

I know that things like hot dogs at a cinema and burgers from the 'dribbly man' in the burger van outside a nightclub don't have a label on them either, but clearly this isn't what I mean by 'non-label food'. This type of 'food' is in a category all by itself and I call it 'mystery food' – it's a complete mystery what's in it! It's funny how, when you see the 'dribbly burger van man' before going into a nightclub, you wonder, 'How can anyone eat that rubbish?' A few drinks later and you're queuing up at 2am to get hold of some. Such are the mind-bending powers of alcohol! I would advise steering clear of 'mystery food' at all times.

Ala Chapman – Super Juice Me

'Thank you for the programme Super Juice Me! programme Jason. My Partner and I completed the 28 days detox and it has transformed both our lives and our perception of food – "real food". My taste buds has reached a higher state – Real food taste more real and processed food tastes less and less real. Literally I can taste the impurities of processed foods. My sense of smell also has increased – now I understand what pregnant women mean "about strong smells" during their pregnancy.'

CAN YOU FIND IT ON AN ISLAND?

A good friend of mine, Jon Gabriel, a guy who dropped over 200lbs eating no-label food and drinking no-label juices, eats and drinks by a very similar principle to 'no-label'. Jon has one question for the people he coaches to eat well: 'Can you find it on an island?' If you can find it on an island then you are good to go. If you can grow it, fish it, or hunt it – it's *no-label* and the body will recognize it. You cannot, for example, find MSG or HFCS (high fructose corn syrup) on an island!

IT'S ALL ABOUT LOW H.I.

I no longer use the term 'no-label food' and instead apply, what I call, 'Low H.I.' principles to the vast majority of what I eat and drink. Like, 'no-label', low H.I. is incredibly easy to understand and is almost impossible to argue against. Low H.I. stands for 'low Human Intervention'. In other words, no matter what the food or drink, all you are looking for is how much has a human interfered with it. The more it's been interfered with, the worse it tends to be. Simple! An orange picked directly from a tree for example is '*no* H.I.', but something like a heavily processed refined sugar- and fat-laced muffin is '*high* H.I.'. We need to understand that *only* wild animals eat nothing but no H.I. foods. To do the same, we'd also have to live in the wild and have skills like Bear Grylls in order to survive. Luckily we don't need to eat no H.I. in order to be slim and healthy. The body can deal with a certain amount of just about *anything* and still stay healthy. If you think back to the GOLD FISH BOWL chapter, we have an inbuilt filter system, which is the reason why, after smoking two to three packets of cigarettes a day, drinking shed-loads of alcohol daily and eating crap from morning till night, I am still here! If I had carried on I honestly feel I wouldn't be here today, as the body can only deal with a *certain amount* of anything, not the bucket-loads that I was pouring in. What this illustrates is that, if you have a cheeky cappuccino, for example, you won't get ill or die! However, we do need to make sure that the *vast majority* of what goes in our body is *low* H.I. if the filtration system is to work efficiently and if we are to have the luxury of being human with no adverse effects.

What I love about the low H.I. way of life is that it doesn't matter if you're a vegetarian, vegan or otherwise. Low H.I. applies to *any* no-label food: fruits, vegetables, grains, nuts, seeds, and lean proteins. This gets rid of the usual nutritional arguments, which can take up days of your life, such as whether you should eat meat or have dairy. My mission is not to turn anyone into a vegetarian or vegan. If you choose to go down that route, feel free. If you think about it, you've been a vegan now for 28 days and you may wish to continue. Equally, if you don't think vegetarianism or veganism is for you, don't become one.

The key to the low H.I. way of eating and drinking is simply to think about what you are about to eat or drink and ask yourself, 'Is it low H.I.?' If you are going to eat meat, at least make sure it's low H.I., for your sake and the animal's. Was it reared organically and did it have natural food throughout its life? If that's the case, it's low H.I., if not it isn't. If you're eating honey, is it low H.I.? Some honey has been interfered with by humans so much it's no longer a natural, low H.I. sweetener. Locally grown honey, as close to what nature intended, is what you're looking for. If you're going to have milk, then is it from an organic, grass-fed dairy? Nothing is really out of bounds, as long as it's a low H.I. version.

Bread is a really good example of just how far removed from nature a food product can get. You can get *very* high H.I. bread, and you can get good low H.I. bread. In terms of nutrition they are worlds apart from each other. The vast majority of bread on sale in supermarkets is loaded with sugar and chemicals. It's nothing more than sugar in your bloodstream and a bloated lump in your stomach. However, flat breads – like pumpernickel and German rye bread – are low H.I. You are looking for bread that's as close to the grain as possible and with the least human interference.

It doesn't matter whether you call it no-label or low H.I., or whether you prefer to think about if in terms of whether or not you would find it on an island. These are all essentially the same thing. We need to make sure the vast majority of what we consume is as close to nature as possible, whilst allowing ourselves the freedom to be human.

THE JAPANESE RULE

There is a principle in personal development known as 'modelling'. Instead of trying to reinvent the wheel, you find someone who is already getting the success you want in a certain area – health and weight loss, in this case – and then you simply follow what they are doing. In other words, do what they are doing and you should reap the same rewards. With the 'Japanese rule' you can go much further and model an entire nation.

There are flaws in modelling just one person. One person's results can be different to another person's results, but if you look at Japanese people as a nation, they're worth modelling. A recent study showed that the Japanese have the longest life expectancy for both men and women and the lowest incidence of degenerative disease of any nation on earth. To put some perspective on this, men in the US were ranked 29th in the world, in terms of life expectancy, and US women 33rd! This is ironic, when you think that, according to Forbes, the US will spend over $3.8 trillion annually on health care this year. The UK also didn't make it to the top 10, despite the billions spent on the NHS. According to the study's findings it was diet which, above all else, had the largest bearing on the statistics. The researchers looked at Japanese people's intake of fermented foods and foods rich in omega-3 and came to the conclusion that these must play a large part in their health and longevity success. Now I have no doubt that what the Japanese eat plays a massive role in why they live so long, disease free, but I feel that an even more important clue lies in *how* they eat.

The Japanese live by an eating principle known as *hara hachi bu*, a phrase which roughly translates as 'eat until you are eight parts (out of 10) full' or 'belly 80 per cent full'. As of the early 21st century, Okinawans in Japan, through practicing *hara hachi bu*, are the only human population to have a self-imposed habit of calorie restriction. On average they consume 1,800-1,900 calories a day and have the highest concentration of centenarians (people over the age of 100) on earth.

'EIGHT PARTS OF A FULL STOMACH SUSTAIN THE MAN; THE OTHER TWO SUSTAIN THE DOCTOR.'
– HAKUUN YASUTANI

I'm not a calorie person. The whole calorie model is flawed. In reality it's not just the number of calories, it's the quality of the calories that counts. However, a great deal of research has been done on food restriction and has shown, time and time again, an increase life expectancy. So, if you like to eat a lot, the message is clear, eat a little less now and you'll live longer and so ultimately get to eat a lot more!

By applying what I term as the 'Japanese rule' of *hara hachi bu* to whatever you eat, it will go a long way to keeping you on the road to optimum health. What you eat is clearly important, and low H.I. is the way to go wherever you can, but how you eat is just as important. However, it is much easier to apply the Japanese rule of *hara hachi bu* to low H.I. foods than to high H.I. foods. High H.I. foods containing loads of refined fat, salt and sugar are often created in a laboratory and are designed to be addictive and to have no natural cut-off point. The advertising slogan of Hobnobs chocolate biscuits perhaps sums it up best : 'One Nibble & You're Nobbled'! It is *much* easier to leave the table at 80 per cent full after eating fish and salad than after gobbling fish and chips.

Natural food, low H.I. food, superfood, non-label food, found-on-an-island food – or however you like to term it – doesn't cause a disproportionate surge in insulin production. It is only when insulin levels are lowered that a person can feel satisfied, which is the main reason why the Japanese rule is much easier to apply with low H.I. foods than high H.I. foods. Low H.I. food doesn't tend to cause a sudden spike in blood sugar – with the knock-on effect of increased insulin production. High H.I., on the other hand, does tend to do this.

There will of course be times when you eat high H.I. here and there, and you can still adopt the Japanese rule. Yes, it may be harder to do this, but if you reach about 80 per cent full and wait 20 minutes, you should feel 100 per cent full. It usually only takes about 20 minutes for the signals to go from the stomach to the brain and for the insulin levels to be lowered.

Even if, for whatever reason, you go back to eating crap (and I sincerely hope you don't) at least give yourself a fighting chance by adopting the Japanese rule for life. Apply this principle on top of a diet most of which is low H.I. and you'll be doing exactly what it takes to *maintain* a healthy and lean body. But please remember to also be human!

THE AFTER-SUPER JUICE ME! OPTIONS

There are, of course, many who would like to know exactly what to do after *Super Juice Me!* To that end, there are many routes you can take. Where you go and which route you choose will heavily depend on your personal situation and where you are on your health and weight journey. If you started your *Super Juice Me!* journey at, say, 300lbs and your ideal weight is, say, 150lbs, then you may well decide to go for the SUPER DUPER JUICE ME! option. Conversely, if you have dropped enough weight, feel great and wish to simply maintain your current weight, then you'll opt for the 80/20 LOW H.I. WAY OF LIFE. If you feel you have more weight to lose, but don't fancy living on nothing but juice for another day, you may go for the J-M-M option.

There are many options to choose from and I do run through them in detail on the app, but for those without the app or DVD here is an overview of …

YOUR TOP TEN OPTIONS

AFTER SUPER JUICE ME!

Choose wisely...

16

OPTION 1:

SUPER DUPER JUICE ME!

This is for people who are seriously overweight and don't wish to stop just yet. The *Super Juice Me!* plan has been devised so that, theoretically, someone who is overweight could continue it every month until they reach their ideal weight. It is, as far as I'm concerned, a much better option than bariatric surgery or chemical 'food' shakes. There is plenty of insoluble and soluble fibre, good fats, amino acids, vitamins, minerals and good carbohydrates on the plan, so repeating it isn't an issue. Please also keep checking in with your doctor and continue to get your stats checked. However, if you are in your stride and want to do another month or two, then simply repeat, and 'Super Duper Juice Yourself'. I have known a few people take this option and had incredible results – there are some good examples in the centre colour pages of this book. Always remember that you have your

Hunger SOS to fall back on any given day too. If you do have a lot more weight to lose, you feel 'in the zone' and have good momentum, then go with this option. Once you have either lost the amount of weight you want to lose, or you come to a point where you feel you've had enough of living on juice only, simply come back to this page and pick a follow-on option that suits your needs at that time.

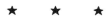

OPTION 2
THE 5:2:5 PLAN

This is designed for those who still have weight to lose, but not as much as those who need Super Duper Juicing. For example, if you were say 60lbs overweight and you dropped 30lbs during *Super Juice Me!*, then this may be the perfect follow-on. This involves juicing for 5 days (usually Monday to Friday) and eating at weekends. The food at weekends should primarily consist of low H.I. foods. You repeat this until you hit your weight or health goal and then move onto a more liberal approach, like the J-J-M, J-M-M or 2:5:2 (explained further on).

OPTION 3
THE 5:2 JUICE DIET

This is a take on the famous 5:2 diet and, I feel, is almost the most perfect maintenance plan. On the original 5:2 diet you eat whatever you like for five days, but for two days a week you restrict your intake to just 600 calories a day, regardless of what constitutes those 600 calories. By doing this you effectively reduce your weekly calorie intake by around 25 per cent, which is a lot.

My version of the 5:2 plan is to eat *primarily* low H.I. foods for five days a week (allowing for a cheeky 'being-human' something here and there!) and have two days of pure juices. If you have four thin juices a day for those two days, you'll be hitting around 600 calories a day. As I've said, I'm not a huge fan of calories as a measurement of diet or health, but for this purpose calories are relevant. The two days *do not have to be consecutive.* Just as many people opt for a Monday and a Wednesday as choose a Monday and a Tuesday. It's your call.

I would say that, of all the maintenance plans, this is a great option. You have just done 28 days on nothing but juice, so two days a week will seem a breeze. There is also good solid scientific evidence backing up two days a week on just 600 calories. And if those calories are coming from nutrition-rich juices, you've got a very good plan for the future. It is proving so popular that we now have this 5:2 option as part of our www.juicemasterdelivered.com service. We have done the maths and devised 600-calories-a-day juices for two days a week. What's neat is that you can order a couple of months' worth, freezer space permitting, and you're all set. I'm not a calorie fan, but people like science and the science has been done on this number, so I've gone with it. I have also been doing this myself and it really has worked a treat!

I have also put together a *5:2 Juice Diet* app, which helps to make it easier as there's a large selection of 600 calorie juices on there. Go to the App Store, put in Jason Vale and it should pop up.

Many want to know the science behind the plan, so I am also doing a small e-book.

OPTION 4
THE 2:3:2 JUICE FLEXI-DIET

Here's a new one. Those who really need a lot of flexibility will probably love it. It's a plan designed to maintain weight loss, supply good levels of nutrition whilst also allowing for a total blow-out if you really feel the human need for it! It's all very well thinking that everyone who does the *Super Juice Me!* plan will be cleaner than clean for the rest of their lives, but, being human, the reality of normal life soon comes home to roost. This is why I have developed this option, for the human inside all of us. It's quite simple:

- **2 days of pure juice**
- **3 days of low H.I. living**
- **2 days of ANYTHING you like!**

How this usually goes is: Monday and Tuesday on four *thin* juices or three *thick* juices a day (600 calories). Wednesday, Thursday and Friday on low H.I. food, usually consisting of juice for breakfast, salad for lunch and protein and salad or veggies for dinner. Saturday and Sunday, eat whatever the hell you want. This, funnily enough, usually still consists of a juice for breakfast –because you are so used to it and almost crave it – a no-rules lunch, consisting of anything, and the same for dinner. These are also the two days when you can have a glass or three of wine, if you want to. You then clean up again on Monday and Tuesday, balance out on Wednesday, Thursday and Friday, and enjoy the weekend with your friends however you see fit. This option really works for a lot of people. It keeps them slim, gives enough nutrients and yet allows the freedom to be human. For many, it's the perfect balance and the one they choose above the rest. It also means you're not constantly picked on for being cleaner than clean and can join in with fellow humans.

★　　★　　★

OPTION 5
THE J-J-M PLAN

By the time most people finish the *Super Juice Me!* plan they are so used to having a juice for breakfast that anything else would seem alien and heavy. This is why most people, even when they know they can now have anything they want on the morning of day 29, still tend to choose a fresh juice. Most then still choose a juice for lunch and have a meal in the evening.

This, I must say, is pretty much how I live my life at least 5 days a week, when I am not doing juice-only cleanses. I find this helps to maintain my weight and keep my energy high. However, I am me and you are you. We are all different, we all thrive on different approaches and all lead different lives. I tend to do this five days a week and have a great deal of food flexibility at weekends, as that's the time I tend to socialize, see friends and go to restaurants. In fact, I am sure that some of the people I know are convinced I never actually juice or eat live food, because they only time they see me is at weekends! My meals in the week tend to low H.I., like hot fish on a bed of salad, but at the weekends *almost* anything goes. (Mind you, you'll never see me walking into a McDonalds, for example, unless I need a pee!) This gives me the freedom to be human. After all, we don't want to get too obsessive about juicing and let it take over our whole lives. That happened to me once for four years, and I am surprised I had any friends left at the end! The five-days-a-week *Juice-Juice-Meal* plan is an option which many choose, but again, it's your call, and I'm just throwing out some suggestions here. It's different for everyone.

★   ★   ★

OPTION 6
THE J-M-M PLAN

I think you already know where I'm going with this one. It's *Juice-Meal-Meal*. However, the meals should be low H.I. where possible, not high H.I., like burger, fries and apple pie! Juice for breakfast, salad or soup for lunch, whatever you fancy for dinner – usually a protein-rich meal, such as avocado salad with a nice piece of fish, or whatever floats your low H.I. boat.

OPTION 7

THE 'TURBO-CHARGE YOUR LIFE' PLAN

My *Turbo-Charge Your life In 14 Days* book was actually written *before* my first juice-only diet book, *7lbs in 7days Juice Master Diet*, yet it has become the follow-on option of choice when people finish that particular juice plan. It is also an option here. It is a 14-day plan, but includes food! There are loads of recipes and it's a kind of pick-and-mix in terms of what recipes suit you. You'll even find my version of fish'n'chips in there! These recipes aren't like those in the *7 Minute Meals* and take slightly longer, but for those who want a specific follow-on plan so they don't have to think for themselves, then *Turbo* is a good option. The *Turbo-Charge Your Life* plan is also now an app. If you have the *7lbs* app, it can be downloaded as an 'in app' purchase, or as a stand-alone one. Unlike all my other apps, there aren't any videos, just the plan and recipes, but it's been priced accordingly. It's a book as well. I fully realize this sounds like an 'up-sell' but it's just an option, there are nine other options to choose from!

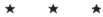

OPTION 8

THE 80/20 LOW H.I. PLAN

Relatively self-explanatory this one. Eighty per cent of what you eat should consist of low H.I. foods (all explained in previous chapter, including ratios) and 20 per cent can consist of whatever takes your fancy. What you'll most likely find though, as I have already touched on, is that what will actually take your fancy after the *Super Juice Me! 28-Day Challenge* will be low H.I. foods anyway. Often people are on 100 per cent low H.I. when they finish the challenge, as their taste buds and cravings have changed so much. Having said that, it doesn't usually take that long before other cravings start to rear their heads again. If this happens, and as long as they don't make up more than 20 per cent of what you consume, you are free to tuck in. Once again, it's just an option and there is no need to start measuring exactly what you are eating in order to work out the exact 80/20 ratio – if you do that you really won't have a life or any friends! Be flexible, clearly, and use it as a rough guide. One thing I have found is that you can usually tell by what's in your shopping basket whether you are adhering to the *80/20 Low H.I. Plan.* You also need to remember that the vast majority of people don't get anywhere near 50 per cent, so if you hit 80 per cent low H.I. a day, you'll be way ahead of the game and flying!

OPTION 9
LIVE BY THE 'HALLE BERRY' RULE!

This isn't so much a plan, but more of a rule you can apply to your life, if you so choose. This doesn't have as much flexibility as low H.I. living. With low H.I., you can eat anything providing it's Low Human Intervention. This is a strict rule where the *only* sugars ever to enter your system are those contained in fruits and vegetables. Although it has become fashionable to knock the sugars in fruits and vegetables of late and for some to claim they are the same as the sugars in a Coke, let's not buy into that myth. I think it's fair to say the obesity epidemic is not being caused by people eating too many apples and downing too much broccoli and beet juice! It is, however, being caused by the over consumption of *refined* sugars, the type you find in sodas, muffins, chocolate, and so on, not the type you find in a pear. Halle Berry once said that the way she keeps in shape is by applying this one strict rule: get your sugars (or carbohydrates if you prefer) only from fresh fruit and vegetables and their juices. This not only means no 'sweets' (or candy, if in the US) but also no bread, pasta and the like, as they turn to sugar in the bloodstream.

As I say, this particular option will certainly not be for all. Many of us – and I'm one of them – cannot contemplate life without the odd bit of warm bread or homemade pasta, but there is no question that, if you *can* adhere to this and are happy to do so, it's *highly* effective.

OPTION 10
THE 'SMALL BUT OFTEN' OPTION

This approach has been used by many over the years and has been in plenty of health and fitness books, usually in conjunction with a weight lifting programme of some kind. I remember reading Bill Philips's *Body For Life* many years ago, in which he advocated six small meals a day, rather than the usual three square meals a day we have all been brought up on. There is a lot to be said for this method. Many people tend to blindly over-stack their plates, especially in the evening, and consume much more in one go than the body requires. This excess tends to get stored, usually as fat. We don't often need anywhere near the amount of food we tend to consume in one meal, but we rarely know this and often feel it's necessary to maintain our energy.

Now I realize I am speaking to the converted at this stage. You've just finished the *Super Juice Me! 28-Day Challenge* and you know first hand just how little fuel we can thrive on. However, here's a good example to illustrate it further. Have you ever been out at a restaurant for dinner and finished your starter but had to wait an age for the main course? If you have, you will know that the longer you wait after you've finished the starter, the more your appetite starts to diminish. When the main dish finally arrives you are angry with the restaurant because you're not hungry any more. This is because it takes a little while before the 'thank you, I've been fed' signals go from your stomach to your brain. We often don't wait for these signals to reach and so we overeat as a consequence. As I mentioned in the previous chapter, if we applied the Japanese *hara hachi bu* approach to eating, we'd naturally eat small portions and stay naturally slim, like the Japanese.

Having said that, though, it's unfortunate to say that the 21st century fast food culture has also infiltrated Japanese shores, and obesity, diabetes and the like are making more and more of a showing.

Please remember with any of the above, there are no hard and fast rules and we are all very different in terms of what works for our particular lives. I have laid out these options as a rough guideline for how to maintain what you have already achieved. The key really is to think 'low H.I.' and to adhere to the 'Japanese rule' wherever possible. This alone will do you well.

YOU DON'T WANT TO SPEND YOUR ONE AND ONLY LIFE TRYING TO EXTEND YOUR LIFE ONLY TO MISS YOUR LIFE IN THE PROCESS!

The idea behind *Super Juice Me!* is to help you take control of your health and to help remove any food addiction problems you may have had. It is essentially 28 days to reset your mind and body, so you can move forward with a sense of freedom and control. The idea is to *remove* a food problem, not to simply move a food problem, and this is the final point I'll make. I know quite a few 'raw fooders'. Raw fooders are people who, like wild animals, only eat raw food. I have had many discussions with people who live by this rule and what I noticed was that a large proportion got into raw food because they had an issue with food. They decided to go 100 per cent raw in order to remove a food issue, but, as I have observed, all that some of them have done is to *move*, not remove, their food issue. Their entire life is now dominated by everything to do with raw food. They often spend every day looking for ways to make sure they live longer. But you don't want to spend your one and only life trying to extend your life only to then realize you missed your life in the process!

Clearly not all raw fooders are like this. David Wolf, perhaps the most famous raw food guy, lives on 100 per cent raw food, but it's *part* of his life. It isn't his *entire* life! He's very happy being 100 per cent raw and lives accordingly. However, there are many in that raw-food world who constantly beat themselves up when they don't hit 'perfection' that day; they drive themselves cuckoo with trying to make raw food dishes which resemble the cooked food they once loved and *still* miss. They often spend a great deal of their life in a state of deprivation and have a constant tug of war going on in their heads. This is not freedom around food and, in my opinion, isn't a healthy way to live. Mental stress can produce a more negative effect on our health and immune system than a latte and, unless you find a balance you are happy with, you are in danger of never truly being free and always trying to play the unwinnable 'perfection game'.

As mentioned, where you go from here and what you do is your call, but whatever you choose I would advise this: do whatever it takes to reach your ultimate goal and then design a regular way of life that works for you. Design something that allows you to stay in great shape and remain healthy, whilst at the same time allowing yourself the freedom of being human from time to time. Choose any of the above suggestions or create a hybrid of them that can fit your world. Whatever you choose to do I wish you well on your journey and if you have had incredible results on this plan, I ask just one favour of you, please, please, please...

JUICE IT FORWARD!

And help to make a juicy difference

17

Nothing inspires others to change more than real people getting real results. You will have probably already seen that some people around you, even those who were not exactly enthusiastic about what you are doing, have started to get the juicing bug purely through seeing the change in you. It is almost impossible not to 'Juice It Forward', as your enthusiasm and results alone will cause a ripple effect. However, what I ask is just one simple favour to help spread the juicy word and to help people begin to take control of their own health: please encourage whoever crosses your path to watch *Super Juice Me!* the movie. By the time you read this, the film will be everywhere, from Hulu.com to Amazon Prime, meaning that for most people it will be essentially be free to watch. All the links will be on www.superjuiceme.com.

THROW A SUPER JUICE ME! PARTY!
AND HELP TO CHANGE SOME LIVES

The reason I ask you to try and get people to watch the film above all other means of Juicing It Forward is because I believe the film has the most impact. I honestly believe you cannot watch the film without being inspired to take a degree of control over your own health. I also know that, while many won't sit down and read a book, most will watch a film.

To help ensure those you care about watch it and take control of their own health, I encourage you to throw a SUPER JUICE ME! party. When the film was first released we made it available to watch for free for one week, and over 500,000 people watched it during that time. I encouraged as many people around the world as possible to throw a SUPER JUICE ME! party. Get as many friends and family members as you can who, you feel, would benefit around to your house to watch the film. At the same time, make a load of fresh juices from the plan and have a SUPER JUICE ME! party. Most people throw these on a Sunday. In much the same vein as Super Bowl Sunday in the good ole US of A, they are referred to as SUPER JUICE ME SUNDAY!

It's your call clearly and just an idea, but they are a great way of helping to Juice It Forward and to make a difference. You just never know the potential impact you could have on someone's life by simply throwing a little SUPER JUICE ME! party and getting them to try some juice and watch the film. Here's a tiny clip from just one email that has come in; it illustrates just what an effect doing this can have. The full letter is in MORE JUICY STORIES TO HELP INSPIRE just after this, but I am hoping this clip might tip you over the edge and get you to throw that party!

'… At my wits end I decided one night with my partner to watch the video. Little did I know that night was going to change my life forever!! 3 months since and I have done the 28 days of juicing and I am now on the J J M. When I last weighed myself I was 78kgs and today I managed to fit back into my size 11 jeans. I have never felt more alive. I love myself like I never have before. I have heaps of energy and believe it or not I don't crave sugar AT ALL. I have more vegetable in a day than I had in probably a year before I started juicing. Snacks now consist of chickpeas fruit and seeds. My dinner now consists of organic natural ingredients and lots of vegetables. To those that are wondering if you should do this or not I highly recommend you give it a go you will not be disappointed I promise! Jason and Team let me raise my juice to you and say thank you for changing my life. You have saved me in more ways that you will ever know …'

Like I said, this was just a small segment from the letter. You can read the full one in the next bit, but you can see the effect the film can have. This is why I ask you to Juice It Forward and help to make a difference.

If, for whatever reason, they're not tempted to join the party and watch the film, pass them this book and tell them to flick to the middle, glossy pages and to read all of the testimonials in the book. That should do the trick! In fact, part of me wonders why I needed to write the whole book at all. I was tempted to simply fill the whole thing with stories of people who had completed the *Super Juice Me!* plan. I have just now been reading a load of them; for some people that will be all the convincing they need!

You can catch me personally on twitter @juicemaster or on

Facebook www.facebook.com/superjuiceme so come say hi!

Thank you in advance for helping to Juice It Forward and, in case our paths never cross, suck the juice out of life – we only get one.

Love Juice – Love Life!

MORE JUICY STORIES

DESIGNED TO INSPIRE!

18

Read them over and over again during the *Super Juice Me! 28-Day Challenge* ... especially on a dark day. They will inspire you to do whatever it takes to continue and complete it, so you can reap the many, many, many rewards that lay ahead!

DROPPED 35LBS / BLOOD PRESSURE BEST IT'S EVER BEEN/ NO HEART PALPATATIONS OR PANICK ATTACKS, INNER FOG GONE!

4 years ago (aged 43) I was diagnosed with heart arrhythmia, it would be sporadic, barely beating, rapidly beating or a mixture of both! This was dealt with 18 months later by having a heart ablation operation to burn off the offending twitching nerves. I was unable to do any real exercise from diagnosis because of possible stroke or heart attack repercussions so, a more sedentary lifestyle began. After the operation and a mini stroke my heart was back to normal with the odd palpitation and panic

attack. My dilemma, no gym would touch me because of heart surgery. So, 2 years passed and I gained nearly 2½ stone (35lbs). I thought that's was that until my pal Kelly told me to watch the 'Super juice me' film. The next day I totally cleared out my fridge/freezer and my cupboards. All bare, no canned stuff/treats/microwave meals. There was nothing! I downloaded the app and bought a £30 juicer from Argos and the first 3 days fruit and veg.

So, myself and Derek...(the juicer, we were in this together!) and my mate Kel at the end of the phone got down to business. I never bothered with the rescue banana or naked bars, once your heads in the right place and as a musician the temptation of beer, snacks, junk food gave me more strength to see the month through and victory...**29 days later, the victory? (a) 2 stone weight loss (28lbs) (b) my blood pressure is the best it's ever been (c) my blood stats are all back to normal since before op (d) no heart palpitations or panic attacks (e) psoriasis showing signs of reducing (f) never had so much energy (g) saved 100's of £'s having not signed up for 12 month gym membership and all my old clothes fit me again from 4 years ago!!!**

What have I learnt? The value of what food does for me, and against me. How it cures me, how it energises me, how it cleanses me, my senses are alive again and best of all, the inner 'fog' has gone!

K. Leitch

WEIGHT LOSS: 15LBS OFF MEDICICATION

Day 26 for me. **Wanted to lose 15lbs and not have to take my meds ever again! My wish has come true. Watching Jason's video today on how to proceed from here.** Very, very rewarding!

J. Thomas

A WHOLE NEW LEVEL OF FEELING GOOD

I've been Super Juiced! Yesterday was day 28, and I have felt very energized and incredibly happy. **I've always been a positive person, but this is a whole new level of feeling good. I actually catch myself saying things like 'I love my life," and "I am so happy!' for no particular reason. And this is while actually I am dealing with some sad things, working two jobs and raising 3 kids on my own.** I take thermos' of juice to work and have managed really well. I thought I was healthy and slim when I started but wanted more focus and energy, but actually now that I feel how good I can feel, I realise I was actually a little run down and feeling overwhelmed. **I don't want to lose this feeling and will definitely keep juicing, and eat even more consciously than before (I was a vegetarian to start with, and thought I ate pretty well except for the occasional bit of total junk!).**

I loved the app I bought with the shopping lists and all the inspiration you give and your charming blend of coach, best friend, comedian and extremely knowledgeable Juice Master. I like it so much I would really consider doing the therapy course. I actually work in public health and my colleagues were in an uproar about my not eating and convinced I was harming myself. I would like be able to be to explain more clearly why that just wasn't so, but I think my energy and enthusiasm will go a long way toward convincing them that I did myself nothing but a very good service.

W. Winn

YOU HAVE SAVED ME IN MORE WAYS THAN YOU'LL EVER KNOW

THANK YOU, THANK YOU, THANK YOU. You have truly changed my life. I was on a spiral down hill heading towards the bottom at a speed that scared me more than I ever cared to admit. I had gone from being fit and a size 10-12 (although now I look back I can see I was never healthy). I can't pin point where I went wrong and I have a lot of excuses but somewhere along my life journey I derailed. A first it was only a kilo here and there. Not to worry weight watcher will fix that. Sure enough I lost the weight and thought "great" now I can go back to living. But yet again the weight slowly started creeping back on. This very quickly became my life putting on weight with a half ass attempt at trying to remedy it with cutting out something I loved. Now for those that know me I have NEVER eaten vegetables. I hated the things I was a sugar addict through and through. I am embarrassed thinking back at what I used to eat. I had deluded myself into thinking what was healthy and what wasn't. Breakfasts were an up and go followed by a large hot chocolate with a caramel shot and a white chocolate and raspberry muffin. The lunch I made was never eaten and my work mates and me went and got lunch, which were normally an ice chocolate, hot chips and a cake. Afternoon tea was what ever I could find that was sweet and if I didn't have anything at home I would make something or go and buy something. Dinner was normally meat and potatoes covered in some high sugar processed sauce then ice-cream for dessert. I could bore you with all the detail but for those that are on this journey you will know what its like to hate looking at yourself in the mirror or how you fell. I hit 96kgs and woke up one day realizing I was almost 100kgs!!! I tried being really good and managed to get down to 91.2kgs when I came across food matters posting the documentary for super juice me. **At my wits end I decided one night with my partner to watch the video.** Little did I know that night was going to change my life forever!!! 3 months since and I have done the 28 days of juicing and I am now on the J-J-M. When I last weighed myself I was 78kgs and today I managed to fit back into my size 11 jeans. I have never felt more alive. I love myself like I never have before. I have heaps of energy and believe it or not I don't crave sugar AT ALL. I have more vegetable in a day than I had in probably a year before I started juicing. Snacks now consist of chickpeas fruit and seeds. My dinner now consists of organic natural ingredients and lots of vegetables. To those that are wondering if you should do this or not I highly recommend you give it a go you will not be disappointed I promise! Jason and Team let me raise my juice to you and say thank you for changing my life. You have saved me in more ways that you will ever know. Here's to the very exciting future.

CHOLESTEROL LEVEL DROPPED TO A HEALTHY LEVEL. EYES BRIGHTER, SKIN BETTER, HAIR SOFTER AND MOOD LIGHTER.

I have just been super juiced...I started the 28 days straight after juice academy and did use some SOS packs especially around day 17 but have completed day 28 yesterday just as the world begins the big summer detox. **I have lost a total of 11 inches from my body, and dropped almost 2 dress sizes, but that is nothing compared to how I feel. I am sleeping better and mower soundly, and the body is happy with 6-7 hours of sleep per night now**...Before even with 8 or 9 hours I woke up tired and lacking energy...haven't woke in the middle of the night since day 2! My eyes are brighter, my skin better, my hair softer and my mood lighter and full of beans. I have more energy than I have had in years and although it took a couple of weeks I am well and truly into the exercise routine now. I have hip bones and collar bones and bones that have been hidden for years but more important than any of that **my cholesterol level has dropped from an unhealthy 7.35 to a very healthy 4.44**... As the world starts a 7 day detox I am starting the launch week of Juice for Life and a life of sheer pleasure and freedom.

T. C. Ward

PARENTS SEEN FANTASTIC RESULTS

My 70 year old dad lost 14 pounds in 3 weeks and has more energy than he has had for years. **My 68 year old mum lost her cough that she had had for 40+ years, which no doctor could diagnose, her constant joint pain, her swollen knuckles and her almost constantly itchy skin. Both my parents' asthma symptoms have reduced massively as well. In 3 weeks!** Just wish there was a retreat like the ones abroad in the UK. Xxx

T. Jones

STOPPED TAKING METFORMIN!

WEIGHT LOSS: 15LBS

Just finished day 28...and starting another 28 days! Feeling so amazing!

I really did enjoy it. **My sugar levels are normal, and I've stopped taking Metformin (yeah!).** I have more energy then I've had in years! I've started cycling in-spite of Fibromyalgia as my muscles and joints don't hurt, so that has increased my activity levels...and **I've lost 15lbs in the process!** I FEEL AMAZING!!!

S. Banks

RE-SET MY MIND TO OVERCOME DECADE OLD PATTERNS

WEIGHT LOSS: 10LBS

Aged 53 and feel 25 on Super Juice Me! Thank YOU for these fabulous lifestyle-altering plans! Simply THE BEST! Day 13 of Super Juice Me, GOING GREAT! App for iPhone BRILLIANT! Simultaneously reading "Freedom From the Diet Trap". EXCELLENT! Your psychology of eating is illuminating. I've learned so much and made the necessary changes and re-set my mind to overcome decade old patterns in only a few weeks! Totally experiencing tremendous benefits – energy, better sleep, strength, amazing skin, peacefulness, genuine JOY, I can feel inflammation reduction daily. Lost 10lbs! So appreciate the extra vid's from BSJD. Jason: your enthusiasm, joie de vive, care for others is totally contagious! YOU are a treasured gift to the world. My husband, George (27 years) & my sons, Jake (19) & Kaleb (15) like the improved me! It is with much gratitude I wish Abundant Blessings to you,

D. Hobel

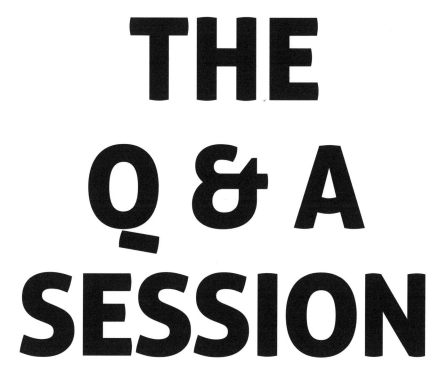

THE
Q & A
SESSION

19

Q: DO YOU JUST HAVE JUICE, OR CAN YOU EAT ANYTHING ELSE DURING THE 28-DAY PLAN?

A: This is a 28-Day *juice-only* plan. Ideally you will consume nothing but freshly extracted, raw fruit and vegetable juices and smoothies, with some special guest thickies added at weekends. *Super Juice Me!* has been designed so your juices are consumed at regular intervals to ensure your blood sugar levels stay stable and you don't get disproportionately hungry. Please understand that, just because you are not using a knife and fork or chewing anything, you are still consuming food. What constitutes food is a combination of key nutritional factors, all of which are in the juices. Most people are over-fed and undernourished. During this 28-day period you can be assured your body is very much being fed. Although the plan has been devised with absence of any solid food, the *Super Juice Me!* plan does have room for a Hunger SOS each day. I have explained this earlier on page 145 in THE TOP TEN TIPS FOR SUPER JUICE ME SUCCESS and in detail on the app. If you do feel hungry, before going directly to your Hunger SOS make sure you are hydrated; drinking a large glass of water can sometimes make all the difference, as we often confuse thirst for hunger. However, if you reach a point where you absolutely must have something or you're going to throw in the towel, then grab your Hunger SOS (a banana, avocado, Juice In A Bar or Simply Nude bar, or some other really good energy bar).

Q: CAN I DRINK ANYTHING EXCEPT THE JUICES, E.G. TEA, COFFEE OR ALCOHOL, WHILE ON THE PLAN?

A: Well...no! You can have as many herbal teas as you like, but normal tea, coffee, alcohol and any other drinks are to be removed from your diet for 28 days. Green tea is OK, for reasons I explained earlier in the book, especially if weight loss is one of your goals. Green tea can aid with this. The only other thing you should and must drink is water; both still and *naturally* sparkling are OK.

Q: I'M NOT A LOVER OF HERBAL TEAS. IS THERE AN ALTERNATIVE?

A: I would recommend you try peppermint herbal tea. Most people tend to like this one. It's worth buying a really good brand, such as Teapigs or Pukka, as they taste amazing. If, however, this isn't for you, then simply cut up some lemon, lime, ginger, fennel or mint, and add boiling water to make your own natural teas.

Q: CAN I CHEW CHEWING GUM WHILST ON THE PLAN?

A: Most chewing gum is made using the synthetic rubber polyisobutylene (which is used in adhesives and sealants, and also as inner tubes for tyres – nice!). Add into the mix some aspartame and various other sweeteners, which are none too kind for the body, and maybe you have your answer? Having said that, there are kinder alternatives on the market, but ultimately if you're doing a detox then it's best to avoid it altogether. Chewing gum also stimulates your gastric juices and makes your body think it's about to be fed, so best left I feel.

Q: I'VE NEVER JUICED BEFORE AND I'M WORRIED ABOUT LIVING ON JUST JUICES AND SMOOTHIES FOR 28 DAYS.

A: Although you are not using your teeth or a knife and fork for the next 28 days, you are still consuming food, just in a liquid form. Living on freshly extracted juices and smoothies is much easier than you might think. Often people are overfed but undernourished, because they are eating processed junk food, which offers little or no nutritional value. By drinking freshly extracted juices your body will be getting a direct hit of nutrition and nourishment and you will be being fed on a cellular level. The real concern is, what will happen if you continue eating and drinking the things that have lead you to the state of bad health you are currently in? This is your chance to clean out your system, improve your health and change your future. Super Juicing isn't for everyone though. If you are too thin, for example, I wouldn't recommend it. Some people need juicing, others need Super Juicing. Make sure you're in the right camp!

Q: I WORK NIGHTS; CAN I STILL DO THE 28-DAY PLAN?

A: Yes of course, however you just need to adapt the times to suit your routine. The *Super Juice Me!* plan is designed so that whilst you are awake you consume your juice or smoothie every three or four hours to keep your blood sugar levels stable and ensure you don't get hungry. If you work irregular hours you can just adapt to fit in with your lifestyle.

Q: DOES IT MATTER IF I DRINK THE FOUR JUICES IN A SET ORDER OR CAN I SWAP THEM AROUND? I WOULD RATHER HAVE THE THICK JUICES DURING THE DAY AND THE THIN ONES IN THE EVENING.

A: The majority of people prefer to have the thickies for breakfast and dinner, which is why the plan is set out in this way. However if you prefer to have them a different way around, that's entirely up to you, as long as you consume the four intended for each day on that day. Please remember though I have designed the plan this way because it's important to get those good fats and amino acids into your body first thing to help regulate your appetite for the rest of the day. It is much easier to do the plan in the way it is set out, rather than trying to switch things around. Fat helps to regulate the appetite and one of the reasons for having the thickies at morning and night. You sleep for around eight hours a night, so the need for a thickie is more in the morning and evening. As mentioned, it's up to you, but it has been designed this way for very good reason, so why mess with it?

Q: DO YOU HAVE TO FOLLOW THE JUICE TIMES LAID OUT FOR YOU OR CAN YOU HAVE THE JUICES WHENEVER?

A: The plan is devised so that you are having a juice or smoothie every three to four hours, to keep your blood sugar levels stable and to stop you getting disproportionately hungry. However, depending on your lifestyle or routine, the gaps between the juices can be tweaked a little, and the start time can certainly be altered. If, for example, you start work at 5am, it is not recommended that you wait till 9am for your first juice. So let common sense prevail and adjust the time of your first juice. Then have your subsequent juices at three to four-hour intervals throughout the day. If you are the kind of person who averages just five or six hours sleep a night, please feel free to add an extra juice each day, if required.

Q: HOW MANY CALORIES PER DAY WILL I BE CONSUMING ON THE PLAN?

A: Although this will vary a little each day, as a rough guide you will be consuming around 1000-1400 calories per day. However, I am not a fan of calories, as they simply don't tell the whole truth. Lets face it, we could all hit our RDA (Recommended Daily Allowance) of calories by munching our way through processed junk food, but it's hardly feeding our bodies. It's far better focus on the nutritional content of what we consume, rather than on the calories. Your RDA of calories should be personal, and not a blanket average, as there are so many different factors to take into consideration: what you are doing on a particular day (physically and mentally), your muscle mass, age, and countless other variables. The recommended RDA for a man is 2,500 calories per day to maintain his weight; for the average woman it's 2,000 calories per day. So, according to this, if a woman were to eat 2,000 calories of refined fat and sugar for days on end and do no exercise, she would supposedly maintain a constant body weight, but in reality I very much doubt that; she would more than likely gain weight. If, on the flip side, she ate 2,000 calories of plant food and fish, the chances are she wouldn't gain an ounce.

Rather than just thinking about weight gain, we need to look at the effect of food in relation to disease. A daily diet of 2,000 calories' worth of processed sugars and fats can be a diet that results in diabetes, heart disease, or high blood pressure. Conversely, a 2,000-calories-a-day diet, made up from fruits, vegetables, seeds, nuts, fish, etc., can create abundant health and vitality and reverse the symptoms of many diseases. If you feel you need an extra juice a day, please add one.

Q: SHOULD I WORKOUT WHILST DOING THE PLAN, WILL I HAVE ENOUGH ENERGY?

A: Yes, I mentioned this in my *Top Ten Tips For Super Juice Me! Success* (page 145). I am a huge advocate of exercise; it is crucial for optimum health, strength and longevity. At our juice-only retreats in Turkey and Portugal, many guests complete up to 5 hours of exercise a day on exactly the same amount of juices you are having on this plan. Some guests are baffled by quite how much energy they have on what appears to be so little fuel. However, the key thing is that you are consuming 100 per cent the right fuel, and it's in a state that your body can easily digest, assimilate and use. Often, digesting the wrong kind of foods robs the body of vital energy, which is why you can feel very tired and lethargic after a big, heavy meal. With juicing, the reverse is true and you liberate that available energy for other activities, such as working out. For the first few days you may feel abnormally tired as a result of the detox process your body is undergoing. You could rest on these days and only exercise if you really feel like it. By day 3 or 4, your 'juicy high' will kick in. You will feel energy running through your veins, and you will be itching to burn it off. that's the time to get those trainers on. It is also vital to keep your metabolism high!

Q: I'VE HEARD JUICING CAN BE BAD FOR YOUR TEETH BUT I REALLY WANT TO DO THE PLAN, SHOULD I USE A STRAW?

A: If the plan was based purely on fruit juices then, yes, this could be a cause for concern and, yes, I would say to always use a straw. However, all of the juices contain fruit and vegetables, so there is a diluted concentration of fruit sugars. It's a good idea to wait at least one hour before brushing your teeth after having a juice. Fruit sugars can temporarily weaken the enamel, but after an hour it will be firm again. If you are still concerned in anyway, then yes use a straw!

Q: IS THERE ANYTHING EXTRA I CAN DO TO MAKE THE 28 DAYS EASIER AND MORE ENJOYABLE?

A: I really advocate feeding your mind as well as your body, so that you are fully submerged in the detox mentally as well as physically. Download and use the '*Super Juice Me!*' app. I really am not just saying this for financial gain; I spent a long time developing the app to make sure it provides the right psychology and coaching to make completing the plan as easy as possible.

My other recommendation is to read a variety of books on nutrition and juicing. And definitely watch the *Super Juice Me!* documentary and others, such as *Hungry for Change* and *Food Matters*. This 'mental juice' will empower you and keep you focused and inspired.

Another thing that really helps is to stop passively watching television. Don't just sit down and aimlessly watch four or five hours of TV each night. Choose what you watch. Until you do a juicing plan or detox, you will be unaware of just how much advertising for food and drink there is and how many food programmes there are on TV. If you watch hours of TV each day, you will be subjecting yourself to the brainwashing and advertising surrounding food, and this will make you mentally crave food. So make life easy for yourself and switch off the box.

And go about your daily life as if nothing had changed. What I mean is, don't lock yourself away from the world for 28 days; there's no need to. Yes, it is slightly odd for your friends and family when you turn up for dinner with a flask of juice, but socializing is about just that, being sociable. It's about catching up, having a giggle and letting your hair down. All you are doing differently is getting your 'fuel' from a different source. If you become a hermit for 28 days, then you really will struggle. There is nothing stopping you going out, meeting friends, going dancing and so on. You just need to adjust accordingly.

Q: CAN I COME OUT TO YOUR RETREAT WHERE THE FILM SUPER JUICE ME! WAS MADE AND DO THE 28 DAYS PLAN THERE?

A: Yes, but clearly it's not cheap! Ideally, from a financial point of view, it's best to do it at home with the help of all of the coaching videos on the *Super Juice Me!* app. However, if you can afford it, then obviously it is much easier to do this at the retreat. There is no other temptation or distraction, and somebody else takes care of all the shopping, juicing and washing up. All you need to do is drink the juice, perhaps participate in some yoga or fitness classes, swim in the pool, jump in the lake, catch some sun, or relax in the spa.

I have done what I can to make this option as affordable as possible and we are having special *Super Juice Me! Juice Camp* months at the retreat so that everyone is in the same boat. That way, people can share a room and bring the price down. I am also looking into the possibility of opening a specific *Super Juice Me!* Juice Camp somewhere in the world, where the only programme on offer would be the *Super Juice Me!* programme. Check out the www.superjuiceme.com website from time to time for more details. Or at the time of writing this book, you can check out www.juicyoasis.com too.

Q: WHAT ABOUT THE FIBRE, SURELY I NEED THIS?

A: All of the juices contain soluble fibre in the form of pectin that effectively forms a type of gel and sweeps through the intestine. Also the daily thickies are blended with whole fruit in the form of avocado or banana or seeds. The 'specials' also contain almond pulp in the milk. It's worth knowing that fibre cannot penetrate the intestinal wall; it does not directly feed the body. All your digestive system does is to extract the juice from the fibre, and then the fibre is excreted from the body. You only need a small handful of insoluble fibre a day to keep things moving, so to speak, which you are getting every day on the plan. To put your mind at rest, I'm going to put the following in capitals and bold, such is the confidence I have in the statement:

YOU WILL GET ENOUGH FIBRE ON THE SUPER JUICE ME! PLAN

Q: DON'T WE NEED CARBOHYDRATES IN OUR DIET?

A: Yes we do. We are so used to thinking of carbohydrates as bread and pasta that many people do not realise that all fruits and vegetables are in fact also carbohydrates. The best carbohydrates on earth! Carbohydrates are a combination of carbon, hydrogen and oxygen. However, I like a play on words, and carbo-HYDRATE is what sets fruits and vegetables apart from complex carbohydrates. Fruits and vegetables are extremely hydrating and consist in *all* cases of at least 70% water. We have over 30ft of intestinal tract which resembles the U-bend you'd find under your sink for waste. It is designed for high water-content fuel, such as fruits and vegetables, which can deliver the nutrients where they are needed in super-fast time and, at the same time, help to flush out any waste. Ironically, on the *Super Juice Me!* plan, the vast majority of what you are consuming are pure *carbohydrates*.

Q: WHERE WILL I GET MY CALCIUM AND PROTEIN FROM DURING THE PLAN?

A: This is a question I get asked a lot and it always makes me giggle a little. When people live on a diet consisting of nothing but crap food, they never stop to ask such a question, but as soon as they go on a juicing plan they become concerned that it might not be nutritionally balanced.

The easiest way to set your mind at rest is to look in the wild at some of the magnificent animals, such as the elephant, horse or giraffe. None of these animals eat meat; they all live on green plants and grass only, and they all have tremendous muscle mass, strength and large teeth (and even tusks). If you think about it, the tusks of a bull elephant are the strongest teeth of any mammal on earth. Don't quote me on that, but it's safe to say they're very big, very solid and very strong, all without a mini Babybel cheese in sight! Calcium is to be found in abundance in green vegetables; it's is also found in many fruits and other vegetables. Protein is synthesised from amino acids, which can also found in all fruits and vegetables. If you are really concerned and don't want to lose any muscle mass, then please feel free to add spirulina, hemp or pea protein powder to your smoothies. All of these are superb forms of plant-based protein. Making sure you do some resistance exercise during the plan will also help.

Q: HOW MUCH WEIGHT CAN I EXPECT TO LOSE?

A: This will very much depend on how much weight you need to lose. Most people will normally lose on average 1lb per day – if they need to lose this amount of weight, that is – so you could expect to lose 28lbs (2 stone) over the 28 days. Please note this happens when you add in the exercise element as mentioned in the *Top Ten Tips For Super Juice Me Success* (page 145). You will always see your biggest weight lose in the first week, when people can lose between 7lbs and 14lbs on average. Your weight loss will then slow down and become more constant and gradual with most people losing between 3lbs and 6lbs in the second week and 2–4lbs in the third and fourth weeks. However, if you don't need to lose 28lbs, then you won't. Also remember that on a regular 'calorie controlled' diet the average weight loss is just 2lbs a week. This is worth remembering if you get to the end and have 'only' dropped 14lbs.

Q: I'M DOING THE PLAN FOR REASONS OTHER THAN WEIGHT LOSS AND I DON'T ACTUALLY WANT TO LOSE WEIGHT. WHAT CAN I DO?

A: This is a tricky one, as 98 per cent of people will lose weight on the plan, but you can reduce the amount of weight loss by adding half an avocado to your second and third juices each day, essentially making them all thickies. The other thing you can do is to include an additional smoothie from the Specials every day, eat one or two bananas each day and snack on plain almonds. If you add to the plan in this way, then you will minimalize weight loss. If you are very concerned about weight loss then add a large avocado salad each day and feel free to add some additional protein to it such as some cooked wild salmon or the like.

Q: COULD I GAIN WEIGHT WITH THE PLAN?

A: This really does depend on your starting weight, compared to the weight you should be. If you are hugely underweight, then the chances are that the plan will provide you with more nutrition and calories than you may normally consume on a daily basis. What's more, the juices and smoothies provide the body with bio-available nutrition in the most easily absorbable state, so if you are underweight because you are not absorbing the nutrition from the food you are eating, then juices and smoothies are incredible. We recently had a nine-year-old girl on our retreat; she was tiny and she drank juices and smoothies and ate an additional banana. She gained 3lbs in the week. (The age limit on the retreats is now 14, just in case the thought that the retreat is full of children is putting you off coming.)

I would suggest you supplement the plan (see the question

above) and, if you really are underweight, then, yes, you could gain weight on the 28-Day plan. Being underweight is often a much bigger issue than being overweight, so please talk to your doctor about this, as there may be an underlying issue here.

If you are overweight and you gain weight during this plan, there is one and only one explanation – YOU DIDN'T DO THE PLAN! Sounds harsh, but I know this subject. I've done it for 15 years. I even had a woman write to me to say she did the seven-day juice plan and gained weight, so I challenged her. I invited her to my retreat and said if she didn't lose at least 7lbs in the week I'd pay for her retreat myself. She lost 11lbs! If you are overweight and you live on juice for 28 days, you will never, ever gain weight. If you hear anyone saying the plan didn't work for them and that they gained weight on it, know one thing – they are telling porkies!

Q: SHOULD I WEIGH MYSELF EVERY DAY?

A: No, I really don't recommend that you become a slave to the scales or that you allow a man-made object to dictate your state of happiness. Trust me, you will *know* that you have lost weight and more than that you will feel and notice a bundle of other benefits from improved energy levels, better sleep and clearer skin, to sharper thinking. If you are really obsessed by a made-up number then I recommend to only weigh yourself at the end of each week.

Q: I LOST A LOT OF WEIGHT IN THE FIRST WEEK BUT NOW I'M STAGNATING, IS THIS NORMAL?

A: This is perfectly normal. In the first week your body drops all kinds of toxicity and retained fluids. It's like 'pulling the plug' of a bath filled with dirty water. After the initial loss you will be losing more fat than anything else. This is a slower process, but a more significant one and you will probably lose around 2–4lbs per week in your third and fourth weeks, depending on how much you have to lose. As you get closer and closer to your ideal body weight, you will lose less and less weight per week.

Q: SHOULD I MAKE ALL MY JUICES IN THE MORNING OR THROUGHOUT THE DAY?

A: You can do it either way, depending on your routine, but fresh is always best, if you possibly can. You can, however, make all your juices in the morning and store them in metal flasks, bottles or 'boosters' in the fridge, to be consumed throughout the day. The plan has been devised so that your first and last juice are the same, and your second and third juices are the same, so you could make juices 1 and 4 in the morning and then juices 2 and 3 together. Personally, I would make juice 1 at the time of consumption, and when it's time to make juice 2, I would also make juice 3 and store it in the fridge. Then I would make juice 4 in the evening, so that I have something to do instead of cooking, and the juice will be fresh. Fresh juice always tastes best. All options are explained in the Top Ten Tips For *Super Juice Me! Success* (page 145).

Q: HOW DO I STORE MY JUICES?

A: Make your juice, pop it in a flask or booster – making sure you fill it right to the top to remove any oxygen and so slow the process of oxidation – and seal it straight away. Then put it in the fridge and drink it within the next eight hours. If you're on the move, get yourself a little cool bag and some freezer blocks. This will also help to keep your juice in tip top condition. Remember, though, that with every hour that passes the juice loses more and more nutrients, so drink it as soon as you can.

Q: CAN I FREEZE MY JUICES TO SAVE TIME?

A: As mentioned above, fresh is always best. But in practical terms not everyone has time to do this so, yes you can. When you freeze juice you lose a little of the nutrient content and some juices will taste 'flat'. For optimum results you need to make your juices in a slow, masticating juicer and blast-freeze them to retain maximum nutrition. This is what we do for *Juice Master Delivered*.

Once you've made your juices, pop them into a BPA-free water bottle or flask, remembering to leave a little room spare for freezing expansion, and then pop them in your freezer. You should then take out a day's worth of juice the night before and store them in your fridge for the next day. It's best to remove each juice about an hour before you want to drink it to ensure it's fully defrosted. If you invest in a Fusion Booster (or similar), this marvellous little gadget allows you to effortlessly freeze your juice, as the actual blender acts as a drinking bottle and you can simply detach the blender flask, pop the lid on and put it directly in your freezer.

Q: CAN I MAKE THE JUICE THE NIGHT BEFORE FOR THE NEXT DAY?

A: I would recommend you make all your juices fresh. However, yes, you could make the morning one the night before, but ensure it is stored in an airtight flask in the fridge. If you make your juice in a fast, centrifugal juicer, then it needs to be consumed within eight hours. However, if you use a slow, masticating juicer, depending on the actual juicer, your juice can be good up to 24 hours later. Low induction, or 'Fusion' juicing is somewhere in-between.

Q: WHEN I MAKE JUICES FOR THE DAY WHAT SHOULD I USE TO STORE THEM IN?

A: You should use a good quality, airtight, dark, metal flask. Sigg do a great range, but other flasks are available, of course. We have a variety available at www.juicemaster.com.

Q: ARE THE RECIPES IN THE BOOK FOR ONE PERSON?

A: Yes, the recipes are designed for one person, so you just need to multiply the recipe by however many people you are making juices for.

Q: SOME OF THE RECIPES MAKE MORE THAN OTHERS, IS THIS NORMAL?

A: Because produce from this country and from around the world varies in size at different times of year, the quantity of juice yielded will vary. This will also depend on the type of juicer you are using. If your juice comes up a little short, please simply add some extra cucumber or an apple. If it is a little over, then lucky you!

Q: WHAT CAN I DO WITH ALL THE LEFTOVER PULP? IT SEEMS SUCH A WASTE.

A: Please don't see this as wasteful. It's only the fibre and this would simply have come out of you anyway. Fibre does not penetrate the intestinal wall, it simply moves through your intestines and comes out as waste. You can, however, use the pulp from juicing as a nutritious face pack or give it to the birds or other animals.

Q: WHAT ABOUT ALL THE SUGAR? ISN'T IT BAD FOR YOU?

A: Sugar is finally receiving the bad press it deserves. Unfortunately, however, fruit sugar is being tarnished with the same brush as white, refined sugar. The sugars are simply not the same, and if you use your common sense, you will appreciate this. Science may say otherwise, but if all sugars were the same, then people could switch chocolate for an apple without any problems.

Think about yourself or someone you know who is a real sugar head – who must eat cakes, biscuits, pastries, sweets or chocolate. If you offered them an apple or a piece of pineapple instead, they would soon tell you where to go! 'Live' fruit and vegetable sugars are not the same as white, refined sugars and do not cause the same harm. However, there's no need to worry in any case, as all the recipes are predominantly vegetable-based, with just a little apple, pear or pineapple to make sure the juices and smoothies taste good – pure vegetable juice is an acquired taste. The thickies also have either avocado or banana, and the additional insoluble fibres help to slow down the absorption of sugars into the bloodstream.

You may be interested to know that, when cooked apple juice and live apple juice were tested for their G.I. or Glycaemic Index rating (G.I. is a number associated with each type of food that indicates the food's effect on a person's blood sugar levels), the cooked juice came out as having a high G.I., whereas the 'live' freshly extracted apple juice had a low G.I.

It is also worth pointing out again that I have received many emails from people who no longer have type 2 diabetes after being on this plan and who are carrying on with a healthy lifestyle. This illustrates, I feel, that the sugars in 'live' juice don't have the same detrimental effect as either white, refined sugar or the cooked juice you find in a carton.

Q: CAN I REDUCE THE AMOUNT OF FRUIT IN THE RECIPES?

A: Yes, if you are an established juicer and prefer a more vegetable taste, then feel free to adapt the recipes by reducing the fruit and increasing the cucumber, courgette, etc. Although cucumber is technically a fruit, it's a vegetable fruit and makes for a wonderful juice base, if you feel apple is too sweet for you or you just don't want any fruit sugars at all.

Q: SHOULD I USE ORGANIC PRODUCE?

A: I always recommend organic produce, although I fully appreciate that sometimes this is not possible, due to availability and cost. If it is cost that is prohibiting you, then please think carefully about this decision and think about how much extra it actually costs to buy an organic cucumber versus a regular cucumber? What is it 40p, 45p more? What difference will that saving actually make to your day compared to the difference that organic produce could positively make to your health? Sometimes we need to re-evaluate our priorities. How much do you spend on new clothes or beauty products, or on over-indulgent meals, wine or nights out? Is organic produce really that much more, or could you afford it, if you made health was your number one priority?

Organic produce is superior because it is free from synthetic chemicals, it is not genetically modified, and is grown with very few pesticides or none at all. And it is more nutritious. So you are paying for what you don't get as much as what you do get!

Q: CAN I JUST MAKE ONE OF THE SPECIALS AND REPEAT IT OR DO I NEED TO STICK TO THE PLAN IN RELATION TO THE SPECIALS?

A: If you prefer one on the specials over the others, you can just have that one instead of the other specials.

Q: I'M ALLERGIC TO/DON'T LIKE A CERTAIN FRUIT OR VEGETABLE. WHAT CAN I DO?

A: If you are genuinely allergic, then, clearly, you should avoid whatever it is you are allergic to. But if you have been told you are intolerant to a certain food, don't just assume it is true. There are genuine cases of people being allergic to certain fruit and vegetables, but it is a rarity. If you would still like to avoid certain ingredients in a juice recipe, please use the table below as a rough guide as to what you can use to replace a specific fruit or vegetable. The rule of thumb is to aim to replace it with a similar thing. Having said that, don't just assume you won't like something. Give it a go first. You'll be surprised how great the recipes taste, and everything has been added for a reason, be it taste or nutrition. PLEASE aim to make the recipes as instructed.

Ingredient	Alternative
Almond milk	Brazil nut milk, soya milk or rice milk
Apple	Pear or pineapple
Avocado	Banana with some Omega-3-6-9 oil
Banana	Avocado
Beetroot	There's nothing quite like a beetroot I'm afraid. It's simply amazing for the blood, and you may be surprised to know that it's actually very sweet. You could just try reducing the quantity slightly, so you can get used to the taste.
Broccoli	Spinach
Carrot	Parsnip
Celery	Courgette (zucchini) or cucumber
Courgette /zucchini	Celery or cucumber
Fennel	Ginger
Ginger	Lemon, lime or fennel
Kale	Chard, spinach or spring greens
Lemon	Lime or ginger
Lime	Lemon or ginger
Mixed Berries	Banana or mango
Mint	Basil
Orange	Grapefruit
Parsnip	Carrot
Pears	Apple
Spinach	Chard, kale, spring greens
Turnip	Parsnip or carrot
Tomato	Cucumber
Zucchini	See courgette

Q: CAN I USE COOKED BEETROOT INSTEAD OF RAW?

A: No, it must be fresh and RAW. Trust me on this one, on the taste front you will hate cooked beet juice!

Q: YOU SAY TO ONLY USE GOLDEN DELICIOUS APPLES, BUT CAN I USE OTHER VARIETIES?

A: You can essentially use any variety of apple. However, Golden Delicious are very mild and not too sweet and work well with every recipe. Granny Smith and Cox tend to be very 'tart' and make the whole juice taste bitter, so avoid them, but Pink Lady and Royal Gala work well. Have a play around and find which you like best, but in all the years I've been juicing I've found Golden Delicious to be best.

Q: I USE DIET WHEY PROTEIN BUT YOU RECOMMEND HEMP PROTEIN IN THE RECIPES, CAN I USE WHEY INSTEAD?

A: I recommend for the 28-Day programme you switch to a hemp-based protein powder, as we want you to be dairy free for the duration of the plan. Because it's a dairy derivative, whey protein is controversial. It can certainly affect your digestive system, so switch to hemp for a natural, plant-based protein.

Q: DO I NEED TO PEEL THE INGREDIENTS?

A: For the majority of the ingredients, keep the peel on, as most of the nutrition is to be found either in the skin or just under it. If you have a Fusion juicer, then please peel the pineapple. Oranges must be peeled, although you won't find any in this plan – its worth noting this for the future. Whether to peel lemons and limes or not is a matter of taste. If you like a real zesty kick, then leave the peel on, but if you prefer a milder flavour, then peel. The main thing to be careful of is that you leave as much as the pith (or white stuff) on as possible, as this is where a lot of the nutrition is to be found.

Q: CAN I ADD ANYTHING EXTRA TO THE RECIPES?

A: Yes, within reason. You can certainly add an additional fruit, vegetable or herb, such as extra lime, mint, ginger, coriander or basil, if you like a particular taste. You can also add spices, such as nutmeg, chilli or turmeric, if you want to spice things up or for their additional health properties. For example, turmeric, paprika and oregano have wonderful anti-inflammatory properties, and cinnamon can help lower blood sugar levels in people with type 2 diabetes.

Q: CAN I USE SHOP BOUGHT ALMOND MILK?

A: You could do, but the plan is based on you consuming raw, live nutrition. Anything in a container is pasteurised and lacks a lot of nutrition. The nut milks are incredibly easy to make, and it's important that these are made fresh for maximum nutrition.

Q: I'M ALLERGIC TO ALMONDS, WHAT CAN I DO?

A: You can use either rice milk or soya milk. If you look online, you will find plenty of recipes for rice milk. However, given that you would have to cook the rice, I'm unsure as to how much benefit there is in making your own. So, as long as you make sure that there are no added sugars or nasties, then you can buy this from the shops.

Q: DO I NEED THE SUPERJUICEME! APP AS WELL AS THE BOOK, OR DO THEY JUST HAVE THE SAME INFORMATION IN THEM?

A: The app is not just a replication of the book. There are videos showing you how to make every recipe, and there's coaching each week to keep you inspired throughout the 28 days. On top of this there are four emergency SOS coaching videos for you to lean on at any time during the 28 days, if you are struggling and need some direct support and motivation to keep you on track. I have spent more time developing and filming this app then any other app, as I am truly passionate about getting people 'Super Juiced'. I know that getting the right mental coaching is imperative for success on this plan. Twenty-eight days is a long time to keep focused, and the app will make the difference between success and failure for many.

Q: DO I REALLY NEED A JUICER, OR CAN I DO THE PLAN WITH JUST A BLENDER?

A: It is essential you have a juicer to embark on this plan. This is non-negotiable! You need both a juicer and blender. Most people already own a blender, but always check www.juicemaster.com for what's hot in the juicing market right now. Like smart-phones, this market moves fast and the self-cleaning juicer might even be out by the time you read this. One can but dream!

Q: DO I REALLY NEED A BLENDER OR CAN I JUST EAT THE AVOCADO OR BANANA, ETC.?

A: Technically, you could just eat the items that you would otherwise blend, as your mouth is a 'blender'. However, you will enjoy the plan so much more if you turn your produce into smoothies. If you don't, it's would be like just eating all the individual components of a recipe, instead of actually making the recipe! I seriously recommend investing in a decent blender; it should form an integral part of your healthy kitchen long after the 28 days.

Q: WHAT IS THE BEST JUICER TO BUY, A MASTICATING, 'SLOW' JUICER OR A CENTRIFUGAL 'FAST' JUICER?

A: There are many different juicers to choose from, and the right juicer for you might not be the right juicer for someone else. At the time of writing, I recommend the Fusion juicer, as it fuses the technologies of 'fast' and 'slow' juicers to produce the finest quality juice, but in superfast time. The whisper-quiet induction motor effectively makes it a 'slow' juicer. This important feature means less heat and creates a better quality juice, which will retain its nutritional content for longer. As you will be living on nothing but juice for the next 28 days, it is vital you buy a good juicer. If it's a centrifugal or 'fast' juicer, please make sure it has a wide funnel to make the process simple and quick. If you opt for a 'slow' juicer, please understand that making your juices will be a far more time consuming process, although the juice will be superior. So, research online and make your choice wisely, depending on what is a priority for you, speed and convenience or top quality. Having said that, there will be a 'new kid on the block' available by the time you are reading this. It's the Retro Cold Press juicer. Their strapline is 'Slow Juicing Made Fast' and, from what I gather, they are pretty good and very cool! Visit www.retrojuicer.com.

Q: I SEEM TO CONSTANTLY NEED TO PEE, IS THAT NORMAL?

A: Yes, over the first few days of the detox you will notice you constantly need to release fluids. The reason for this are two-fold: you are consuming around 1.6-2 litres of nutrient-rich fluid per day, which is maybe far more fluid than you normally consume; and cucumber and celery, amongst other fruits and vegetables, are strong diuretics and help the kidneys work efficiently to flush waste and toxicity from the system.

Q: I HAVE NOT HAD A BOWEL 'MOVEMENT' FOR A FEW DAYS. IS THIS NORMAL?

A: Some people go less than usual during the plan and this is to be expected, as the amount of insoluble fibre in your diet has been greatly reduced and there is very little for the body to eliminate. This is nothing to worry about and is perfectly normal. If you feel constipated and in pain, then I would suggest taking some chia seeds or psyllium husks – but be sure to read the instructions – as these pulp up when added to water and form a gel-like fibre to sweep through the intestines.

Q: I HAVE THE OPPOSITE PROBLEM: I CAN'T STOP GOING. IS THIS A PROBLEM?

A: No, this is nothing to worry about. This is often a very good sign, as the body is ridding itself of waste. Things should find a balance after a few days. Once again though, if for whatever reason you feel something isn't quite right, contact your doctor. Things happen in life in general, and you don't want to coincidentally have a health issue come up in the first few days and dismiss it as 'detox'. Always listen to your body!

Q: MY URINE OR POO IS RED. IS THIS BLOOD?

A: The most likely answer is no. This is probably caused by the beetroot. If you believe you are passing blood, then go and see your doctor immediately.

Q: I'VE JUST STARTED THE PLAN, I'M GETTING HEADACHES, AND I HAVE NO ENERGY. IS THIS NORMAL?

A: When your body is detoxing, depending on just how 'toxic' you are, it is quite common to experience headaches and initial energy loss. You need to understand that you were falsely stimulating your body with things like caffeine, alcohol and sugars. Now that these stimulants have been withdrawn, your body is re-establishing its equilibrium and, during this time, you will suffer an energy loss. What you are currently experiencing is your 'true' level of health. However, the good news is that, after two to four days, the headaches should subside; after three to five days, you should start to get a great deal more energy. It is important that if you feel like this, and you are in a position to do so, you rest and sleep to allow the body to use its energy to effectively 'spring clean' you internally.

Q: I'M ON WEEK 3 AND I WAS FEELING AMAZING, BUT NOW I'M FEELING LOW. WHY IS THIS?

A: This is perfectly normal and something to just accept as part of the 28-Day journey. Week 3 is often the toughest for people; this is the week when you have to dig deep and focus on all the reasons why you started the challenge in the first place. This is a great time to re-watch the coaching videos or the emergency SOS coaching videos on the Superjuiceme app.

This is very much like running a marathon or any endurance event; the beginning is easy, the end is filled with elation and euphoria that you have nearly finished, but the really tough part is when you are around the half-way mark.

You may be thinking 'life is too short' and considering quitting, but in the words of the now controversial Lance Armstrong, 'Pain is temporary, quitting lasts a life time.

I agree that, yes, life is too short. It's too short not to be able to wear the clothes you want to wear, to slip on a beautiful bikini or shorts and walk comfortably around the beach, or to throw on your trainers and go running or playing football with the little people in your life. Life is too short to be diagnosed with a serious disease in your 40s or 50s and to be told you need medical intervention for the rest of your 'short life'. So dig deep, spend 5 minutes thinking of all the reasons why you are doing this, give yourself a virtual slap and 'suck it up princess'. In just 7-14 days you will feel like a superhero and will have the biggest sense of achievement and pride.

Q: I'M DOING THIS FOR MY SKIN, BUT ITS ACTUALLY GOT WORSE, WHY IS THIS?

A: It can be perfectly normal to expect your skin to flair up throughout the first 7-14 days. Your skin's cycle is 28 days, so for some people it may take the full 28 days before you see improvements. If you are doing this for psoriasis or eczema, I highly recommend supplementing this plan, as there are some key minerals and essential Omega oils that are vital for healthy skin. Please go to www.juicemaster.com, download the FREE 'Clear Skin' manual and add the recommended supplements.

Q: SHOULD I STOP USING MY STEROID CREAM FOR MY SKIN?

A: Yes, I recommend that you stop applying steroid creams and use only natural shower gels and pure coconut oil as a body moisturiser twice per day during the programme and beyond. Steroid creams only treat the symptom and do not address the cause, so they give short term results, with the side effects of thinned skin and discoloured pigment. If you think of your skin's condition as being like a pan of boiling water over a flame, then applying steroid cream is like adding ice to the boiling water. It stops it boiling temporarily, but does nothing to address the underlying cause.

When you stop using the cream, you must expect to see a flare-up in your skin in the first few days, but remember this is a 28-Day journey and this flare-up will subside. Having said that I don't know your condition, so please always see you doctor before coming off any medication.

Q: MY TONGUE/TEETH FEEL FURY AND I CAN TASTE METAL, WHY IS THAT?

A: Your tongue is an organ of elimination and sometimes your mouth can feel odd as some of the toxicity is being expelled.

Q: I FEEL REALLY EMOTIONAL, IS THIS NORMAL?

A: Many people during the 28-Day detox will experience some form of emotional rollercoaster, from glorious highs to emotional lows. This is perfectly normal. During the plan you will:

1. Not be under the influence of alcohol or refined sugars, both of which create false highs and associated lows. This means your body will have to find its own natural rhythm

once again; during this process you may well feel emotional.

2. Not be using foods and drinks to mask your real emotions and you will free up a lot of time that was otherwise spent shopping, cooking, eating out, getting drunk, dealing with a hangover, etc. This valuable time will no doubt allow you to reflect on your health, your lifestyle, your priorities and your future. It will also allow you to focus on why you need to be 'Super Juiced'. All of this together can manifest in feelings of emotion and upset. This is nothing to worry about and is a valuable part of your journey.

Q: SHOULD I STOP TAKING ALL MY MEDICATION?

A: No. You should only ever stop taking medication with your doctor's approval and supervision. My hope is that, after you complete the 28-Day plan (or even during it) and overhaul your diet and lifestyle, you will be able to get your doctor to retest you and – assuming your condition improves – reduce your medication. For many people the goal will be to improve your health so much that in two, three or four months' time your doctor will advise that there is no need for you to continue on medication.

Q: WILL JUICING HAVE ANY CONTRAINDICATIONS TO ANY OF THE MEDICINE I AM TAKING?

A: As you may imagine, this is a question that is impossible for me to answer, given the hundreds upon thousands of different combinations of medicines you might be taking. So please seek medical advice, depending on your specific medicine, as certain fruits and vegetables do not go with certain drugs.

Q: CAN I DO SUPER JUICE ME! IF I'M PREGNANT?

A: I would certainly recommend that you incorporate juicing into your diet whilst pregnant, as there is no better way of getting key minerals and nutrients into your – and, therefore, your baby's system. However, I would not recommend that you embark on an exclusively juice programme whilst pregnant, as this programme will certainly result in symptoms of detox and weight loss, which is something to be avoided during pregnancy.

Q: CAN I DO SUPER JUICE ME! WHILST BREASTFEEDING?

A: Yes, there is no reason why you shouldn't follow this programme while breastfeeding, as long as you make sure you listen to your body and supplement the plan with extra avocado, banana, yogurt, nuts (as long as you and baby are not allergic) and seeds. You may also feel like you need an extra juice or smoothie here and there, which is to be encouraged.

Q: I'VE GOT KIDNEY PAIN, IS THIS NORMAL?

A: During the first few days of the detox, some people report slight pain in their kidney region. However, if this persists or is more than just mild, I would advise to stop the plan and seek medical advise.

Q: I FEEL SICK AND WEAK AND I'M GETTING STOMACH ACHES. IS THIS NORMAL AND WHAT SHOULD I DO?

A: Nausea is not a normal response to a juice plan, but occasionally some people on juice plans for the first time will feel a bit off-colour. This shouldn't last longer than a day or two, while your system adjusts to the detox.

You may be allergic to a particular fruit or vegetable, or if you have 'Super Juiced' your juices with 'spirulina', 'wheatgrass' or 'Power Greens', you may have an allergy to one of these ingredients. Some people find wheatgrass and spirulina can make them nauseous, as they are nutritionally so potent and your system may not be ready for this level of nutrition. So remove these from your juices, and if you are still feeling nauseous after two days, then come off the plan IMMEDIATELY and see your doctor. It may be due to something unrelated to the juice detox.

Q: I KEEP BEING SICK AND HAVE DIARRHOEA. IS THIS PART OF THE DETOX?

A: No, this is not a natural part of the detox. You should try and consume some water and electrolytes and seek medical advice as soon as possible.

Q: I HAVE FINISHED SUPER JUICE ME! AND FEEL AMAZING. I'D LOVE TO VOLUNTEER AT A RETREAT OR GET INVOLVED WITH JUICE MASTER IN SOME WAY, HOW DO I GO ABOUT THIS?

A: We are always looking for good, genuine people to help our mission to 'Juice The World'. Please write to info@ superjuiceme.com

JUICE THE WORLD!

TWITTER

@juicemaster

FACEBOOK

www.facebook.com/superjuiceme
www.facebook.com/juicemasterltd

WEBSITES

www.superjuiceme.com
www.juicemaster.com

TO YOUR DOOR!

www.juicemasterdelivered.com

JUICE RETREATS

www.juicyoasis.com
www.juicymountain.com

JUICE BARS

www.juicemasterjuicebars.com

JUICE THERAPY

www.juicetherapy.co.uk